Spices:
The Elixir of Life

Edited by
Dr. Amit Krishna De
Ph.D., FICN, FNESA, FAEB

Originals
Delhi-110052

ISBN 13: 978-81-8454-103-8
ISBN 10: 81-8454-103-1

Published by
Originals
A-6, Nimri Commercial Centre,
Near Ashok Vihar Phase-IV,
Delhi-110052
Phone: 011-27302453, Fax: 011-47061936
e-mail: info@Lppindia.com
website: www.Lppindia.com

Printed at
D K Fine Art Press P Ltd.
Delhi-110052

PRINTED IN INDIA

Foreword

I compliment the authors for having collated up-to-date information on various aspects of spices in this book viz. botanical/ horticultural as well as the taste, flavor, medicinal and potential benefits. Certainly the wealth of knowledge available in this book will serve one and all interested in these spices for one reason or the other. The information on their uses and nutrition is of special interest to the health practitioners, dieticians and housewives who will come to know new ways of using Indian and exotic spices with an international perspective.

The editor also has to be appreciated for his efforts, in compiling the book, which will be useful not only to the spice people but also to the research-scientists, horticulturists, entrepreneurs, state officials, administrators as well as students. No doubt this book will be of great help and use to all those interested in chilli, cardamom, fenugreek and other important spices.

Prof. (Dr.) S. M. Paul Khurana
Director, Amity Institute of Biotechnology,
Amity University Haryana,
Gurgaon Manesar 122413
(Former Vice-Chancellor
Rani Durgawati University, Jabalpur).

Preface

Spices have been used since ages in tribal and folk medicines and different traditional forms of ancient medicine like Ayurvedic, Unani and Sino-Tibetan systems. In Ayurveda specially, spices contribute a major amount for the treatment of major disorders of the body and are officially recognized as a drug material in the pharmacopoeia of several countries like India, China , USA and Europe. They are used as carminatives, antiseptics or musking the unpleasant taste of drugs. Homoeopathic medicine has been using spices as one of the major ingredients in most of their preparations. In this respect, some major spices like chilli, pepper, ginger, garlic, bishops weed, cumin, coriander, turmeric, mustard, asafoetida, fenugreek, onion, fennel, anise, cinnamon, tamarind etc play a major role. Spices were also used in perfumes, offerings, medicine, preservatives, flavours, cultural marks, cosmetics, in perfurmery, soap manufacturing, pecticides, and as condiments. Natural red and yellow colour prepared from red chilli, turmeric and saffron respectively were used as dyes.

Spices are parts of plant such as, roots, buds, flowers, barks, seeds which can be obtained from large number of different plants. The flavouring properties of spices comes from volatile oils and also fixed oils and small amount of resins. Sometimes a blend of different compounds such as alcohols, phenols, esters, organic acids, alkaloids and sulphur contribute to the flavour. Spices also contain the usual components of plant products such as protein, carbohydrates, fibre, minerals and tannins and vitamins. The spices as identified by Spices Board, India is given in Table 1 :

Table 1. Spices available in India

Name	Botanical Name	Parts of Plant
1. Cardamom		
(small)	*Electtaria cardamomum* Linn	Fruit
(large)	*Amomum subulatum* Roxb	Fruit
2. Pepper	*Piper nigrum* Linn	Fruit
3. Chilli	*Capsicum frutescens* Linn	Fruit
4. Ginger	*Zingiber officinale* Roscoe	Rhizome
5. Turmeric	*Curcuma longa* Linn	Rhizome
6. Coriander	*Coriandrum sataivum* Linn	Leaf & seed
7. Cumin	*Cuminum cyminum* Linn	Fruit
8. Fennel	*Foeniculum vulgare* P. miller	Fruit
9. Fenugreek	*Trigonella foenum graecum* Linn	Seed
10. Celery	*Apium graveolens* Linn	Fruit
11. Aniseed	*Pimpinella anisum* Linn	Fruit
12. Bishop's weed	*Trachyspermum anisum* Linn	Fruit
13. Caraway	*Carum carvi* linn	Fruit
14. Dill	*Anethum graveolens* linn	Fruit & Seed
15. Cinnamon	*Cinnamomum zeylanicum* Blume	Bark
16. Cassia	*Cinnamomum aromaticum* Nees	Bark
17. Garlic	*Allium sativum* Linn	Bulb
18. Curry leaf	*Murraya koenigii* Linn	Leaf
19. Komam	*Garcina indica* choisy	Fruit

20. Mint *Mentha piperita* Linn Leaf
21. Mustard *Brassica jaucea* Linn Seed
22. Parsley *Petroselinum crispum* Seed
23. Pomegranate seed *Punica granatum* Linn Seed
24. Saffron *Crocus sativus* Linn Stigma
25. Tejpat *Cinnamomum tamala* Nees Leaf
26. Pepper long *Piper longum* Linn Fruit
27. Star anise *Illicium verum* J D' Hooker Fruit
28. Vanilla *Vanilla fragrans* Ames Syn. Pod
29. Sweet flag *Acorus calamus* Linn Rhizome
30. Greater Galanga *Alpinia galanga* Linn Rhizome
31. Horse radish *Armoracia rusticana* Gaertner Rhizome
32. Caper *Capparis spinosa* Linn Fruit
33. Clove *Syzgium aromaticum* Linn Bud
34. Asafoetida *Ferula asafoetida* Linn Resin
35. Cambodge *Garcinia cambogia* Gaertner Pericarp
36. Hyssop *Hyssopus officinalis* Linn Leaf
37. Juniper berry *Juniperus communis* Linn Berry
38. Bay leaf *Laurus nobilis* Linn Leaf
39. Lovage *Levisticum officinale* Koch Leaf
40. Marjoram *Marjorana hortensis* Leaf
41. Nutmeg *Myristica fragrans* Houttuyn Seed
42. Mace *Myristica fragrans* Houttuyn Aril
43. Basil *Ocimum basilicum* Linn Leaf

44.	Poppy seed	*Papaver somniferum* Linn	Seed
45.	All Spice	*Pimenta dioca* Linn	Fruit
46.	Rosemary	*Rosmarinus officinalis* Linn	Leaf
47.	Sage	*Salvia officinalis* Linn	Leaf
48.	Savory	*Satureja hortensis* Linn	Stem, leaf
49.	Thyme	*Thymus vulgaris* Linn	Fruit
50.	Oregano	*Origanum vulgare* Linn	Leaf
51.	Tarragon	*Artemisia dracunculus* Linn	Leaf
52.	Tamarind	*Tamarindus indica* Linn	Fruit

(Source : Spices Board, Cochin)

Spices are prone to spoilage by insect or microbial attack. Hence, spiceoils containing all the active ingredient of spices are extracted or marketed. This is done by steam distillilation of ground spices. Oleoresins are obtained by solvent extraction of ground spices. Acetone, Isopropanol, Methanol, Hexane etc. are used as solvents. Processed products of spices are convenient to use, free from contamination, have better storage life and easy to transport. In curries, bakery products, pickles, processed meat, beverages, liquors etc. spices are used as flavouring agents varying or enhancing the flavour. Sometimes spices can help mask off the flavour of foods, some spices possess antoxidant properties while others are used as carminatives. Some spices are used as preservatives, others like clove and mustard prevent food spoilage due to their antibicrobial properties. Many spices also possess important physiological and medicinal properties.

Scientists have demonstrated that the same chemical compounds that protect the spiciest spice plants from their natural enemies are at work today in foods from parts of the world where — before refrigeration — food-spoilage microbes were an even more serious threat to human health and survival than they are today. The proximate reason for spice use obviously is to enhance food palatability. Traits that are beneficial are transmitted both culturally and genetically, and that includes taste receptors in the mouth and taste for certain flavors. People who enjoyed food with antibacterial spices probably were healthier, especially in hot climates. They lived longer and left more offspring. And they taught their offspring and others - the ultimate reason for using spices is to kill food-borne bacteria and fungi. Garlic, onion, allspice and oregano, for example, were found to be the best all-around bacteria killers, followed by thyme, cinnamon, tarragon and cumin. Capsicums, including chilies and other hot peppers, are in the middle of the antimicrobial pack , while pepper of the white or black variety inhibits 25 percent of bacteria, as do ginger, anise seed, celery seed and the juices of lemons and limes.

Countries with hotter climates used spices more frequently than countries with cooler climates. Indeed, in hot countries nearly every meat-based recipe calls for at least one spice, and most include many spices, especially the potent spices, whereas in cooler counties substantial fractions of dishes are prepared without spices, or with just a few. As a result, the estimated fraction of food-spoilage bacteria inhibited by the spices in each recipe is greater in hot than in cold climates.

Scientific experiments since the late 19th century have documented the antimicrobial properties of some spices, herbs, and their components. Studies in the past decade confirm that the growth of both gram-positive and gram-negative foodborne bacteria, yeast and mold can be inhibited by garlic, onion, cinnamon, cloves, thyme, sage, and other spices. Effects of the presence of these spices/herbs can be seen in food products such as pickles, bread, rice, and meat products. Thus, it is observed that higher levels of spices are necessary to inhibit growth in food than in culture media. Spices that have been shown from our laboratory to have inhibitory effect on various microorganisms includes cumin, cinnamon, black cumin, clove, onion, Bishop's weed (ajowain), chilli, garlic, celery, basil, tejpat, nutmeg, small cardamom, caraway, turmeric, tamarind, aniseed, black pepper, horse raddish, pomegranate seeds, cambodge, mustard, rosemary, thyme, oregano and star anise.

Besides anti-microbial properties, spices also have (i) anti-inflammatory (ii) analgesic (iii) anti-oxidant (iv) anti-obesity (vi) anti – pollutant and (vii) anti-mutagenic properties. Recent studies indicate that capsaicin from chilli, piperine from pepper, gingerone from ginger, curcumin from turmeric , thymol from bishops weed etc have a lot of antioxidant properties. Based on the studies carried out in our laboratory, spices can be grouped according to their iological activities and medicinal properties. These properties of spices justify their traditional uses in various folklore and ancient medicines in different cultures as customs. Some of these properties are given in Table 2

Table 2 Biological properties of some spices

Biological properties	Spices
Cholesterol lowering:	garlic, onion, fenugreek, turmeric, chilli, pepper
Hypoglycemic:	fenugreek, onion, garlic, cinnamon
Anti-oxidant:	turmeric, chilli, pepper, clove, ginger
Anti-inflammatory:	chilli, turmeric, ginger, mustard, clove, cardamom
Anti-mutagenic:	garlic, mustard, turmeric
Digestive:	fennel, chilli, bishops weed, mint, onion, fenugreek, turmeric, anise, asafoetida, coriander, dill, ginger, ovage, marjoram
Anti-microbial:	turmeric, asafoetida, anise, basil, hyssop, sage, thyme, chilli, cumin, bishops weed, star anise
Anti-obesity:	chilli, pepper, ginger onion, garlic

Anti-ulcer:	chilli, pepper, ginger, bishops weed
Analgesic:	chilli, pepper, ginger, clove, ginger
Anti-asthmatic:	chilli, onion, pepper, ginger

Results indicate that spices have dual type of action showing inflammation, pain, heat, redness and swelling on acute treatment and anti-inflammation, analgesia, anti-microbial, antioxidant and anti-mutagenic actions on long term treatment. Recent studies indicate that spices at low dose are beneficial for human health. Hence, spices may be the main natural source of therapeutic agents in near future. Medicines from such a cheap source as spices which are consumed daily may help to shape the future health of mankind.

This book entitled :Spices : The Elixir of Life" is a collection of articles written by eminent scientists relating their research work on spices. This up – to – date data from different parts of the world will help the pharmacists, analysts, botanists, toxicologists, chemists, pharmacognosists and biochemists to learn more about the important properties of major spices. The book focuses on the medicinal properties as well as health benefits of some important spices that are daily used in our diet and also deals with some aspects of cultivation. Students, teachers, researchers, growers of spices and medicinal and aromatic crops, practitioners of traditional herbal medicine and commercial houses selling spices and manufacturing drugs from natural ingredients, will find this publication very useful.

Amit Krishna De

List of Contributors

Anita Doeve
Department of Agricultural, Food & Nutritional Science
University of Alberta, Edmonton,
Alberta, Canada

Asim K. Duttaroy
Department of Nutrition, Institute for Basic Medical Sciences,
Faculty of Medicine
University of Oslo, POB 1046 Blindern,
N-316 Oslo, Norway
Email: a.k.duttaroy@medisin.uio.no

K. Srinivasan
Department of Biochemistry and Nutrition,
Central Food Technological Research Institute,
Mysore - 570 020
E- mail: ksri.cftri@gmail.com

Peter, K.V.
Kerala Agricultural University,
K.A.U P.O.Thrissur 680656
Email:kvptr@yahoo.com

Syed Ibrahim Rizvi
Department of Biochemistry,
University of Allahabad,
Allahabad 211002
E mail: sirizvi@gmail.com

Suaib Luqman
Department of Biochemistry,
University of Allahabad,
Allahabad 211002

Sadhan Kumar, P. G.
Kerala Agricultural University,
K.A.U P.O.Thrissur 680656

Tapan K. Basu
Department of Agricultural, Food & Nutritional Science
University of Alberta, Edmonton,
Alberta, CANADA
Email : Tapan.Basu@ales.ualberta.ca

Indira, P.
Kerala Agricultural University,
K.A.U P.O.Thrissur 680656

Pradeepkumar,T
Kerala Agricultural University,
K.A.U P.O.Thrissur 680656

S. N. Acharya
Agriculture and Agri-Food Canada Research Centre,
Lethbridge, AB Canada T1J 4B1
Email : Surya.Acharya@agr.gc.ca

S. K. Basu
Department of Biological Sciences,
University of Lethbridge,
Lethbridge, AB, Canada T1K 3M4
Email :saikat.basu@uleth.ca

K. Acharya
Deparment of Botany,
University of Calcutta,
Kolkata-700018, WB, India

S. Paul
Laboratory of Expermiental Immunology,
Department of Botany,
Gurudas College,
Kolkata-700054, WB, India

S. Datta Banik
Department of Anthropology,
Vidyasagar University,
Kolkata- 721102, WB, India

R. Prasad
Department of Biological Sciences,
University of Lethbridge,
Lethbridge, AB, Canada T1K 3M4

Pulok K. Mukherjee
School of Natural Product Studies,
Department of Pharmaceutical Technology ,
Jadavpur University, Kolkata-700032,
E-mail: pulokm@gmail.com

N. Satheesh Kumar
School of Natural Product Studies,
Department of Pharmaceutical Technology ,
Jadavpur University, Kolkata-700032,

S. Bhadra
School of Natural Product Studies,
Department of Pharmaceutical Technology ,
Jadavpur University, Kolkata-700032,

S. Ponnusankar
School of Natural Product Studies,
Department of Pharmaceutical Technology ,
Jadavpur University, Kolkata-700032,

R.Basavaraju
Department of Biosciences,
Sri Sathya Sai University Prashanthi Nilayam,
Ananthapur Dist, A.P. 515134.

V A Parthasarathy
Director,
Indian Institute of Spices Research,
P.B. No 1701, Marikunnu,
Calicut-673012, Kerala
E-mail: parthasarathy@spices.res.in

V Srinivasan
Scientist,
Indian Institute of Spices Research,
P.B. No 1701, Marikunnu, Calicut-673012, Kerala
E-mail: srinivasan@spices.res.in

K N Shiva
Scientist,
Indian Institute of Spices Research,
P.B. No 1701, Marikunnu, Calicut-673012, Kerala
E-mail: shiva@spices.res.in

D Prasath
Scientist
Indian Institute of Spices Research,
P.B. No 1701, Marikunnu, Calicut-673012, Kerala
E-mail: shiva@spices.res.in

Contents

Spices: Novel Sources of Antioxidants and their Potential Health Benefits

Tapan K. Basu **and** ***Anita Doeve***

In recent years, potential health benefits of antioxidants have received much attention in medical and scientific communities. Spices that are used in foods as flavouring agents are increasingly being recognized to be novel sources of natural antioxidants. This chapter discusses a select group of commonly used spices with particular references to their antioxidant contents and their potential biological significance. The spices discussed include cinnamon, ginger, turmeric, fenugreek, oregano, basil, capsicum, rosemary, sage, star anise, thyme, nutmeg, cumin and coriander.

Introduction

Reactive oxygen species (ROS) are created through various physiological and biochemical processes such as mitochondrial respiration, the activation of phagocytes, the biosynthesis of endoperoxides by cyclooxygenase and lipooxygenase, the oxidation of various compounds by enzymes such as xanthine oxidase, and the presence of transition state metals such as Fe^{2+} and Cu^{2+}[1,2]. The ROS are known to inflict damage upon cells by promoting the oxidation of lipids, proteins and DNA to induce peroxidation, modification, and strand break. In addition to the reactive species derived from biological processes, humans are also exposed to environmental sources of pro-oxidants such as cigerette smoking, ultraviolet radiation and oxidizing agents. The possible sources of oxidative stress including their mechanism of actions, are shown in Table 1. There are, however, many naturally occurring substances, which function to protect against the potentially harmful effects of pro-oxidants. These substances, termed 'antioxidants' can be defined simply as substances that inhibit oxidation. Antioxidant compounds must be present in biological systems in sufficient concentrations to prevent an accumulation of pro-oxidant molecules, a state known as 'oxidative stress'. The oxidative stress is increasingly being implicated in the pathogenesis of many age-associated degenerative diseases, such as coronary heart disease (CHD), cancer, diabetes, rheumatoid arthritis, alzheimer's disease, and senile cataract.[3]

Table 1. Sources of oxidative stress

Sources	**Mechanism**
Mitochondrial electron transport	Leakage of superoxide ($O_2^{\bullet}$-) as a result of inadequate reduction of oxygen
Transition metal ions	Iron and copper give rise to hydroxyl radical (HO•) formation
Inflammation	Activated phagocytes produce free radical
Enzymes (e.g., xanthine oxidase)	$O_2^{\bullet}$- release due to reperfusion of ischaemic tissues
Drug metabolism	Free radical metabolites produced
Cigarette smoking	Gas phase with concentrated free radicals
Radiation	UV light, x-rays

Antioxidants, such as vitamins C and E, as well as ß-carotene and flavonoids are known to be beneficial against free radical damage and hence the oxidative stress-related chronic diseases. However, the concept of balance is a prerequisite in the field of antioxidants, since antioxidants, when present in excessive quantities, can potentially become pro-oxidants. This hypothesis is perhaps best supported by the study showing a negative effect of ß-carotene supplement on the incidence of lung cancer among smokers,[4] while foods that are rich in ß-carotene along with other nutrient and non-nutrient antioxidants have consistently shown protective effects agaist a variety of cancers, especially the lung (Table 2). The dose-related biphasic effect of α-tocopherol has also been shown on the LDL-receptor activity.[5] Furthermore, the propagation of antioxidant activity of vitamin E has been suggested to be dependent upon the presence of other factors, such as ascorbic acid and selenium.[6] Ascorbic acid, on the other hand, requires cellular thiols such as glutathione in order to be regenerated from its radical form. In view of these reports, it seems that a cocktail of antioxidants is more effective than one individual antioxidant in isolation. In recent years, the potential of antioxidant rich fruit and vegetables to reduce the risk of degenerative diseases has thus gained a great deal of interest in medical and scientific communities. Recently, the Health Canada had revised the recommendation of fruit and vegetables for adults from 5-7 portions to 7-10 portions per day (Eating well with Canada's Food Guide, December 2007).

Table 2. Epidemiological evidence of the protective effect of fruits and vegetables against cancer

Site of cancer	No. of studies	↓ Risk	↑ Risk
Lung	25	24	0
Larynx	4	4	0
Oral cavity	9	9	0
Oesophagus	16	15	0

Stomach	19	17	1
Colorectal	35	20	3
Bladder	5	3	0
Pancreas	11	9	0
Cervix	8	7	0
Ovary	4	3	0
Breast	14	8	0
Prostate	14	4	2

Adapted from Block et al, 1992.

Because of the importance of natural sources of antioxidants, there have been a continuous search for their novel sources of the nutritional factors. In recent years, spices have been increasingly being recognized to be potential sources of natural antioxidants. This article discusses a select group of commonly used spices that could be the most effective sources of antioxidants in our diet.

Cinnamon (*Cinnamomum zeylanicum*)

Cinnamon is a small evergreen tree (10-15 meters tall), belonging to the laurel family "Lauraceae". It is native to Sri Lanka and also cultivated in South America and West Indies. The bark, due to its distinct odor and taste, is widely used as a spice and flavoring material. Its flavor is due to an aromatic essential oil, which is a golden-yellow color, with the characteristic odor of cinnamon and a very hot aromatic taste. The taste and odor come from cinnamic aldehyde (cinnamaldehyde). Its golden-yellow color darkens by forming resinous compounds via absorbing oxygen during ageing. In addtion to cinnamaldehyde, the essential oil extract of cinnamon contains ethyl cinnamate, eugenol, beta-caryophyllene, linalool, and methylchavicol.

The etheric, methanolic and water extracts of cinnamon have been found to be high in total equivalent antioxidant capacity (TEAC), and that this capacity is thought to be contributed by their phenolic content.[7,8] These in vitro results have also been substantiated by an *in vivo* cross-sectional clinical study[9] showing a significant beneficial effect of cinnamon in alleviating the complications of many oxidative stress-induced illnesses. The presence of Type A polymers (water-soluble polyphenolic compounds) have been identified in cinnamon.[10] The protective effect of these antioxidants against oxidative stress-associated metabolic syndrome has been well investigated. These studies have clearly suggested that cinnamon reduces fasting blood glucose and cholesterol levels, increases insulin sensitivity, and modifies body weight in type 2 diabetes.[11-13] The cinnamon intake has also been reported to reduce post-prandial glucose response in association with delay in gastric emptying without affecting satiety in healthy subjects.[14] It is noteworthy that according to a dose-response study the cinnamon at less than 1 g per day for 40 days can be effectively hypoglycemic and hypolipidemic in type 2 diabetes. Such effects seem to be maintained even when the cinnamon intake is ceased for 20 days. These results suggest that a dietary inclusion of cinnamon, even on an irregular fashion, can be potentially beneficial in the management of diabetes.

Cinnamon polyphenols have been found to affect multiple steps relating to glucose and insulin function. Thus, the polyphenols activate insulin receptors by increasing their tyrosine phosphorylation activity and by decreasing phosphatase activity that inactivates the insulin receptor.[15] The cinnamon polyphenols also increase the amount of insulin receptor ß and GLUT 4 protein,[16] increase glycogen accumulation by increasing glycogen synthase activity and decreasing glycogen synthetase kinase-3ß activity,[17] and increase the amount of the early-response of tristetraprolin, which is an anti-inflammatory protein.[18] All these activities point to the fact that the whole cinnamon or its extracted polyphenolic components can be highly effective in decreasing risk factors associated with diabetes and cardiovascular disease and improvements in the metabolic syndrome as a whole.

Ginger (*Zingiber officinale*)

The ginger plant is native to India and China and is now grown in all over the world, particularly in West Africa and Carribian. It is a perennial plant, 3-4 ft tall, producing aromatic, fibrous knotty, buff-colored tuberous rhizomes. The dried and fresh rhizome is used essentially as a spice, but also as a medicinal herb.The rhizome part of ginger contains active components known as gingerols and gingerdione. These constituents seem to have a wide variety of pharmacological properties including diaphoretic, antiemetic, carminative, circulatory stimulant, anti-inflammatory, and antiseptic.[18] Other ginger constituents, such as 6-shogaol and galanolactone, are known to act on serotonin receptors in ileum.[19] The predominant antiemetic action of ginger is localized in the GI tract, but there is evidence that the ginger constituent may also have an effect on the central nervous system. The ginger component 6-gingerol, a phenolic alkanone, has been suggested to have anti-inflammatory effects by inhibiting cyclooxygenase and lipooxygenase pathways.[20]

Ginger is thought to contain antioxidants, which seem to have a free-radical-inhibiting index greater than that of synthetic antioxidant preservatives, such as BHA and BHT.[21] The antioxidant activity of ginger has also been evident by a number of *ex-vivo* and *in-vivo* experimental studies. Ginger has thus been found to inhibit lipid peroxidation in rat liver microsomes.[22] The shelf-life of a variety of meat products has been markedly improved by adding ginger extract, an indicative of its antioxidant effectiveness.[23] Furthermore, pre-treatment of mice with ginger rhizome has been shown to reverse dose-related radiation mediated elevation in the lipid peroxides and depletion of glutathione (GSH) levels in tissues; these results were in parallel with reductions in the radiation sickness and mortality of the animals.[24] Apolipoprotein E-deficient mice are genetically prone to develop atherosclerosis. Feeding a diet containing a standadized ginger extract to these animals resulted in a marked reduction in the development of atherosclerotic lesions, when compared with their control counterparts.[25] This antiatherogenic effect was associated with a significant reduction in plasma total and LDL-cholesterol as well as a marked reduction in the LDL basal oxidative state. These results point to the possibility that an oxidative modification of LDL by the ginger extract may have been accounted for the inhibition of the pathogenesis of atherosclerosis. The inhibition of lipid peroxidation has also been demonstrated in the presence of diabetes, which is also subject to oxidative stress as being a major factor for its pathogenesis.[26] Using streptozotocin (STZ)-induced diabetic rats, feeding a diet containing ginger powder has thus been shown to markedly decrease in plasma antioxidant capacity and red blood cell content of malonaldehyde, reflecting a decrease in lipid peroxidation.

In an attempt to isolate and identify antioxidants from ginger, a group of gingerol compounds substituted with an alkyl group bearing 10-, 12- or 14-carbon chain length were isolated from the dichloromethane extract of rhizomes, using repeated chromatographic techniques.[27] This study has clearly suggested that the substituents of the alkyl chain are important factors for ginger to contribute both radical scavenging effect as well as inhibitory effect of autooxidation of oils. Given the high relative antioxidant activity of ginger rhizome and its evidence-based pharmacological effects in oxidative stress related disorders, ginger should be considered to be a dietary essential.

Turmeric (*Curcuma longa*)

Turmeric is a tropical perinnial plant in thc same family as ginger. It is native to India, and cultivated throughout the tropics around the world. Growing to a height of about one meter, it bears pairs of lance-shaped leaves of alternate sides of the stem. At the base of the stem, there is a knobby rhizome some what resembling ginger, which is the applicable part of turmeric. In addition to its flavoring and coloring properties as well as its popular use in curry, turmeric is also known to have active medicinal components. Thus it contains components that are both anti-inflammatory and antioxidant, making it useful for treating inflammatory conditions.

Its anti-inflammatory activity is thought to be mediated by inhibiting cyclooxygenase-2, prostaglandins and lekotrienes.[28] The major active components with antioxidant property include curcumin and demethoxycurcumin. These compounds are yellow pigments, which are responsible for the color of turmeric spice. The antioxidant activity of the compounds is dependent upon delocalization of the phenolic radical through conjugation of the alkyl chain to the ketone function.[29]

More recently, a heat stable turmeric antioxidant protein (TAP) has been isolated from an aqueous extract of turmeric.[30] Using rat brain homogenate and thiobarbituric acid reactive substance (TBARS), this protein has been shown to be highly effective in inhibiting lipid peroxidation at a concentration of 50 ug/mL, while protecting Ca^{2+} - ATPase activity. The latter was found to be associated with the prevention of loss of –SH groups. Another water soluble antioxidant molecule has been isolated from turmeric, called Tumerin.[31] This is a heat stable noncyclic peptide containing 40 amino acid residues, of these there are 3 residues of methionine which are partly responsible for the antioxidant activity. Tumerin has been shown to be highly effective in protecting membranes and DNA against oxidative injury. ROS-induced releases of arachidonic acid and the mutagenic activity of t-butyl hydroperoxide have also been found to be inhibited by the antioxidant peptide molecule.

3'azido-3' deoxythynidine (AZT) is a drug which delays disease progression in HIV-infected patients but causes many serious dose-dependent side effects (Richman and Andrews, 1988). Turmeric or curcumin have been shown to help to reduce the doses of AZT and hence the drug toxicity when taken together, without compromising the drug's effectiveness in slowing the progress of HIV.[32]

Fenugreek (*Trigonella foenum-graecum L.*)

Fenugreek is an annual herbaceous crop, widely cultivated in Ethiopia and India. It belongs to the Papilionaceae section of the family Leguminosae. Fenugreek plants have an erect growth habit with a height of 0.5 to 0.8 meters, mainly tap rooted with one main stem. Stems have alternating branches up to 0.4 meters with alternating compound pinnate trifoliate leaves 2 to 3 cm long. Flowers are axillary and cream in colour (1 cm long), developing into long slender (15cm) green then yellow-brown pods. Each pod contains 10 to 20 green then yellow-brown seeds with a unique hook like groove. The applicable part of fenugreek is the seed. The seeds have a distictive bitter taste and odor, which is why they are, following grinding, used as spice in food. The fenugreek seeds are also used as a medicinal herb.

Fenugreek seeds contain 23-26% protein, 6-7% lipid and 58% carbohydrate of which 25% is dietary fiber.[33] The seeds have been reported to have hypoglycemic and hypocholesterolemic properties. The unique dietary fiber (galactomannan), amino acid (4-hydroxy-isoleucine) and saponin (glycosidic steroid) contents in the crop, especially in its seeds, are thought to be responsible for these health benefit potentials. According to an *in vitro* study involving sections of small intestine, taken from model rats for insulun resistance (JCR rats), the presence of galactomannan,extracted from fenugreek seeds, markedly diminished intestinal uptake of glucose.[34] The effect was found to be dose-related and that no difference was observed between the genetically determined lean and obese rats. The viscous property of galactomannan was essentially responsible for impeding the in vitro intestinal absorptopn of glucose. These results were confirmed in a metabolic study involving normal Sprague-Dawley rats, which were fed a diet containing up to 5.0 % galactomannan for 4 weeks.[35] The postprandial blood glucose response was markedly decreased with galactomannan. Compared with the control counterpart the animals fed a diet containing galactomannan for 4 weeks had significantly less body weight gain, which was accompanied by a reduction in epididymal adipose weight, reductions in food intake and plasma insulin levels. Furthermore, the galactomannan-fed animals had significantly reduced plasma levels of triglycerides and total cholesterol. Further studies have shown that saponin, extracted from the fenugreek seeds has also the ability to modify cholesterol status by its capacity to bind both cholesterol and bile acids.[36] In addition to galactomannan and saponin the amino acid, 4-hydroxyisoleucine, found in fenugreek has the ability to release insulin through stimulating pancreatic ß cell.[37] Based on these data, it appears that fenugreek has multiple components that have the potential to provide health benefits when included in the daily diet.

The fenugreek seed contains appreciable amounts of zinc and manganese as well as phenolic compounds, flavonoids, carotenoids and coumarins. These antioxidant components are also thought to be the contributing factors toward health beneficial properties of the seed. Polyphenolic compounds, extracted from fenugreed seeds, have been found to scavenge hydroxy radicals and inhibit H_2O_2-induced lipid peroxidation in rat liver mitochondria.[38] These in vitro results were further substantiated by the *in vivo* protective effects of the phenolic extract against alcohol-induced hepatoxicity in rats as determined by their modifying effects on the markers of hepatic injuries, such as liver function tests, alcohol metabolizing and detoxifying enzymes, and cytochrome-c reductase activities.[39] The modifying effect of fenugreek seed on blood lipid peroxidation and antioxidants has also been examined in Alloxan-induced diabetic rats.[40] This study has shown that supplementation with fenugreek seeds markedly minimizes Alloxan –mediated increase in lipid peroxidation, accompanied by increased circulatory levels of ß-carotene and glutathione. The fenugreek seeds following their germination have been found to be highly enriched with antioxidant properties due primarily to the presence of polyphenols and flavonoids.[41]

Based on the available data, it appears that fenugreek seeds have a wide variety of health-promoting activities. Hence, it is important to increase awareness of the public and health professionals as to the unique properties of the spice.

Oregano (*Origanum vulgare*)

Oregano is originally a Medeterranean spice. It is a perennial plant, growing to 20-80cm tall, with opposite leaves. The applicable part of the plant is the leaf and oil. The dried leaf is more often used than the fresh one. Oregano is high in antioxidant activity, due to a high content of phenolic acids and flavonoids.[42] Main antioxidant is the monoterpene phenol known as thymol that has strong antiseptic properties, and its isomer, carvacrol, another antibiotic that acts synergistically with thymol to increase the antibacterial effect of both. The presence of carvacrol and thymol in essential oils from oregano plants, grown wild in Greece, was found to be related to the antioxidant activity as determined by peroxide values.[43] These results were supported by the dose-related inhibiting effects of phenolic acids in ethanolic extracts of clonal oregano on free radical scavenging as well as lipid perixidation capacities.[44] The phenolic acids, due to their antioxidant properties are also thought to have the potential to inhibit growth of *Helicobacter pylori*. Both methanolic and aqueous extracts of dry leaves from oregano have also been found to have the potent antioxidant activities as shown by their abilities to block peroxidation catalysis by iron, neutralize free radicals, and interrupt lipid radical chain reactions.[45]

A number of flavonoids with antioxidant capacities have been isolated from oregano.[46] These include flavone apigenin, flavanone, eriodictyol, dihydroflavonols, dihydrokaempferol, and dihydroquercetin. In addition to these antioxidant factors, appreciable amounts of nutrient antioxidants have been identified in oregon. The four homologues of tocopherol have thus been found to be present in its hexane extract; the tota amount of tocopherol ranged from 288 – 672 ppm.[47]

Basil (*Ocimum basilicum*)

Basil is trully a native plant to India and Iran and other tropical regions of Southeast Asia. It is prominantly used as a culinary herb in Italian as well as in Southeast Asian (such as in Thailand and Vietnum) cuisines. The applicable parts of basil are the above ground plant parts, which are rich in antioxidants. Thus, basil is rich in ascorbic acid and phenolic compounds like methyl cinnamate, methyl chavicol, ocimene, cineole, and linalool.[48] It could potentially constitute important sources of antioxidant phenolics in the diet, providing 125 mg of gallic acid equivalent, and 106-140 mg of ascorbic acid equivalent per gm of dry weight.[49] Basil also contains a wide range of essential oils,[50] which are rich in phenolic compounds and a wide range of other natural antioxidants including polyphenols, such as flavonoids and anthocyanins.[51]

A variety of basil extracts have been found to possess markedly higher free radical scavenging and metal chelating activities than in BHT, BHA, and α-tocopherol, as determined by DPPH scavenging and ferric thiocyanate methods.[52] In this study the antioxidant activities of basil were expressed primarily due to its total phenolic content. Rosmarinic acid seemed to be the predominant phenolic acid in basil. According to the DPHH scavenging assay system, one molecule of rosmarinic acid captures 1.52 radicals *in vitro.*[53] In addition to this free radical scavenging property, basil extracts have also been shown to display an inhibiting effect on lipooxygenase activity.[54] The modifying effect of varying concentrations of basil powder on the lipid peroxidation products of refrigerated (upto 14 days) pork meat was thus examined. The presence of basil resulted in significantly decreased formations of TBARS (thiobarbituric acid substances) and peroxide values as well as conjugated diene and hexanal content of the stored meat; the inhibition of the lipid peroxidation markers was all dose-related to basil powder.

Capsicum: Chilli and Red peppers (*Capsicum annuum*)

The capsicums are represented by many diverse spices and cultivars, including chilies, paprika and red peppers. They are native to the Western Hemesphere and probably evolved from an ancestral form in Bolivia/Peru area. Chilies are considered vegetables when green, a spice when red and dried; botanically they are all berries. The quantities of the various phytochemicals found in capsicums vary considerably between different cultivars. Chilies are particularly very rich in capsaicin, which is the phytochemical that gives plants of this genus their strong flavored irritant effect. Chilies' most recognizable trait is pungency, resulting from a mixture of seven homologous branded-chain alkyl vanillylamides (capsaicinoids), often called capsaicin. The capsaicins are produced in glands where seeds are produced. While seeds are not the source of pungency, they occasionally absorb capsaicin because of their location. Chiles are considered to be high in antioxidants. A green chili can contain Vitamin C six times as much as an orange. One medium sized chili can thus provide 130% of the recommended daily allowance (RDA) for vitamin C; it is also rich in vitamin E and ß-carotene. In addition to these antioxidants, capsicums, as a whole, contain a variety of other antioxidants including caffeic acid, chlorogenic acid, coumaric acid, feluric acid, hesperidin, quarcetin, and rutin.[55] Total antioxidant activity in pepsicum increases as its green pods turn red (Table 3). Because of the high content of a variety of antioxidants, chilie's health potentials have brought renewed interest. Thus, they have been well documented as factors for prevention and treatment of obesity and its associated disorders, such as diabetes.

Table 3. Antioxidant activity in sweet bell peppers[56]

Bell pepper Type	Antioxidant activity* (trolox equivalent, umol/g fresh pepper)
Green	2.1 ± 0.6

Yellow	3.2 ± 0.5
Orange	3.5 ± 0.5
Red	3.9 ± 1.0

*Antioxidant activity was determined using 2,2' – diphenyl-1-picrylhydrazyl (DPPH method).

Obesity occurs as a result of increased energy intake and decreased energy expenditure. Adding chilli or red peppers to meals has been reported to cause modest reductions in appetite and inductions in dietary fat metabolism in healthy subjects.[57] Postprandial studies with meals containing chili in young subjects have also been shown to increase basal metabolic rate (BMR) in association with an increased body fat oxidation.[58] It is of further interest that in a group of non-diabetic subjects, a chili-blend diet (30g/d) intake for 4 weeks decreased C-peptide and insulin secretion, and increased hepatic clearance of insulin, as evidenced by a higher C-peptide/insulin quotient.[59] These results may have implications in the control of postprandial hyperinsulinemia.

Overall human studies point to the concept that capsaicin (chilli) facilitates appetite control and body weight stability. There is, however a need for more clinical observations to document that the beneficial metabolic effects do apply to post-obese individuals, who have to maintain a loss of body fat. It is also important to point out that a maximum tolerable dose may be necessary to have an inhibitory effect of chili on fat intake.[60] The strong pungency of capsaicin is often a limiting factor for many not being able to tolerate chili for loosing/maintaining body weight. It is, however, noteworthy that there are non pungent capsaicin analogues (capsiates), derived from a non-pungent cultiver of *Capsicum annuum*, and that this variety has been shown in mice to have similar effects as capsaicins on the oxygen consumption (VO_2) and hence energy expenditure.[61] More recently, similar results were obtained in human subjects with obesity-categorized BMI scores.[62] Thus, an intake of non-pungent capsaicin analogues for 4 weeks enhanced $VO_{2,}$ resting energy expenditure and fat oxidation, making the non-pungent analogues to be potentially useful for weight reduction.

Other commonly used spices

In addition to the spices discussed above, there exist a number of other spices with antioxidant activities and potential health benefits (Table 4).

Clove (*Eugenia caryophylleta*)

Traditionally, clove is used for GI tract problems (e.g., flatulence, nausea and vomiting) and as a flavoring in food, beverages and cigarette. These potential uses are thought to be due to its content of gallic acid and eugenol, the potent antioxidants.[63] In effect, eugenol comprises upto 90% of clove oil. The antioxidant activity of clove is evident by the fact that it increases storage life of butter cakes for more than 4 weeks by protecting them from rancidity.[64] Clove, especially its oil has been found to be antiaggregatory, and inhibitor of cyclooxygenase and lipooxygenase reflecting their potential as an antioxidant spice.[65]

Table 4. Some commonly used spices including their active antioxidant components

Spice	Botanical name	Active components
Clove	*Eugenia caryophyllata*	Eugenol, gallates
Rosemary	*Rosmarinus officinalis*	Rosmarinic acid, rosmanol, camosic acid, camosol
Sage	*Salvia officinalis*	Carnosol, camosic acid, rosmanol, rosmarinic acid

Star anise	*Illicium verum*	Protocatechuic acid
Thyme	*Thymus vulgaris*	Thymol, carvacrol, flavonoids, p-cuene-2,3-diol
Nutmeg	*Myristica fragnans*	Myristic acid, eugenol
Cumin	*Cuminum cyminum*	Diphenyl Picrylhydrazyl (DPPH)
Coriander	*Coriandrum sativun*	DPPH

Rosemary (*Rosemarinus officinalis*)

Rosemary is a perennial plant, native to the Mediterranean region. Apart from being used as a spice, rosemary has the potential to be a crop of phytochemical significance. The penolic compounds in its essential oil express high antioxidant activity. Antioxidant properties of several polyphenol skeletons, isolated from rosemary, have been characterized.[66] These include phenolic diterpenes (e.g., carnosic acid, carnosol, and 12-O-methylcarnosic acid), caffoel derivatives (e.g., rosemarinic acid), and flavones (e.g., genkwanin and isoscutellarein 7-o-glucoside). Rosemary extracts containing these antioxidants seem to have antibacterial and antifungal properties as well as they have been shown to enhance nerve growth and possess radioprotective effects against chromosomal damage in human lymphocytes.[67]

Sage (*Salvia officinalis*)

The applicable part of sage is the leaf and volatile oil. Sage contains 1-3% of volatile oil that may be responsible for pharmacological activity, which include antidepressant, antiinfammatory, anticholinesterase, and estrogenic.[68] A number of antioxidants found in rosemary have also been found in sage; these include rosmarinic acid, carvacrol and luteolin . Many of the pharmacological effects of the sage may be potentially mediated by its antioxidant contents.[69]

Star anise (*Illicium verum*)

The applicable part of star anise is the seed, which contains volatile oil, 75% of which is anethole.[70] Star anise is a common spice widely used in Asian countries. It has also been used in traditional medicine as stomachic, carminative, and expectorant. Aqueous and ethanolic extracts of star anise have been found to have antioxidant activity. Protocatechuic acid was isolated from star anise as a compound mainly responsible for scavenging activity against DPPH radical.[71] The antioxidant activity of protocatechuic acid was further shown by its inhibiting effect on the Cu ion- and peroxy radical-induced oxidation of isolated human low density lipoprotein.[72]

Thyme (*Thymus vulgaris*)

Thyme is a basic ingredient in French, Greek, Italian, Arabic and Carribean cuisins. It contains thymol, carvacrol, flavonoid, and p-cynene-2,3-diol constituents. These antioxidants are thought to be responsible for the antispasmodic, antitussive, and expectorant effects.[73] Rosmarinic acid seems to be the predominant phenolic compound in thyme as in sage and oregano.[74] The total antioxidant activity in thyme oil has been shown to be markedly greater than that in BHA or tocopherol.[75]

Nutmeg (*Myristica fragnans*)

Nutmeg is a large evergreen tree, native to Indonesia. In effect, it produces two spices – nutmeg and mace. Nutmeg is the seed kernel and mace is the seed coat (arillus) that separates the seed from its outer husk. Nutmeg seeds contain 20-40% of a fixed oil, commonly called nutmeg butter. This oil contains myristic, stearic and palmitic acids.[76] Nutmeg also yields 8-15% of an essential oil, containing myristicin, eugenol, and safrol. Other isolated compounds in the oil include a variety of phenolic compounds.[77] Among the isolated phenolic compounds, Eugenol has been found to have antioxidant activity in an appreciable level.[78] Using methanol extract of nutmeg an in vitro study has also shown to have an inhibiting effect on NO production as well as NO scavenging potential.[79]

Cumin (*Cuminum cyaminum*)

It is a member of the parsely family (belongs to the family Apiaceae), a native plant from East Mediterranian to Indian subcontinent. Cumin's distinctive flavor is due to its essential oil content, the main constituent being cuminaldehyde (4-isopropyl-benzaldehyde), which has been shown to scavenge superoxide anion in vitro.[80] Cumin seeds also contain flavonoids and are thought to inhibit the induction of gastric squamous cell carcinoma in mice.[81] Chemopreventive effects of cunib cyminum in chemically induced forestomach and uterine cervix tumors in murine model systems. Using rat liver microsomal lipid peroxidation and DPPH radical scavenging methods, an appreciable amount of antioxidant capacity was found to be present in a variety of cumin.[82]

Coriander (*Coriandrum sativun*)

It is also known as cilantro belonging to the parsely family, a native plant to Southestern Asia and West to North Africa. Coriander seems to be high in both carotenoids and phenolics . In addition, coriander leaves are rich in caffeic acid, ferulic acid, gallic acid and chlorogenic acid.[83] The presence of these antioxidants was found to reflect on the in vivo antioxidant capacity, as determined by their inhibiting effects on both plasma and liver lipid peroxidation in rats.[84] Overall, coriander leaves seem to possess stronger antioxidant activity than the seeds, and the ethyl acetate extract contributes more antioxidant capacity than any other fractions of either leaves or seeds.

Conclusion

A spice is often defined as any part of a plant that is used in a diet for its aromatic properties. In recent years, however, spices are increasingly being identified as important sources of various phytochemicals. They are thus valuable sources of phenolic compounds, which seem to have better antioxidant properties than nutrient antioxidants, such as vitamins C and A, and carotenoids. Some of the phenolic compounds, present in spices, have been shown to exhibit even a better antioxidant effect when mixed with other plant compounds than when used separately. Spices exhibiting strong antioxidant capacities have been essentially evolved from *in vitro* studies, suggesting their significant role in increasing shelf-life of foods. It is important that *in vivo* studies are carried out to determine the clinical importance of the in vitro findings in the body, especially in relation to their medicinal claimes. In effect, there have been hardly any well designed clinical trial to support spices' therapeutic claims or their effective dose levels. Herbs are generally considered to fall under the category of "generally recognized as safe", but only when they are used in foods as flavoring agents. In view of our growing interest in the medicinal potential of spices because of their high antioxidant properties, more evidence-based studies are warranted to determine their efficacy, effective dose levels, contraindications, drug-spice interactions, and other toxicities.

References

1. Halliwell B) **44**: 6-13. (1996).

2. Yucan YV and Kitts DD Endogenous antioxidants: role of antioxidant enzymes in biological system. In: Shaihids F (ed). Natural antioxidants: Chemistry, Health Effects and Applications. AOCS Press, Champaign, Illinois, pp. 258-270. (1997).

3. Thompson KH, Godin DV *Nutr Res* **15:** 1377-1410. (1995).

4. Goodman GE, Thorrquist MD, Balmas J *J Natl Cancer Inst* **96:** 1729-1731,(2004).

5. Pal S, Bursill C, Bottema CDK, Roac PD (1999) Regulation of low density lipoprotein receptor by antioxidants in human health and disease (eds. Basu TK, Temple N, Garg M). CAB International, Oxford.

6. Park DV (1999). Nutritional antioxidants and disease prevention: Mechanisms of action. In Antioxidants in Human Health and Disease (eds. Basu TK, Temple N, Garg M), CAB International, Oxford, pp. 1-13.

7. Mancini-Filho J, Van-Koiij A, Mancini DA, Cozzolino FF, Torres RP. *Boll Chim Farm* **137:** 443-447. (1998).

8. Shan B, Cai YZ, Sun M, Corke H. *J Agri Food Chemistry* **53**: 7749-7759, (2005).

9. Ranjbar A, Ghasmeinezhad S, Zamani H, Malekirad AA, Baiaty A, Mohammadirad A, Abdollahi M. *Future Medicine* **3**: 113-117. (2006).

10. Anderson RA Diabetes Care **26:** 3215-3218. (2003).

11. Blevins WL, Gutierrez-Williams CM, Klugar WJ, Coleman CI *Diabetes Care* **31**: 41-43. (2008).

12. Chase CK, McQueen CE. *Am J Health Syst Pharm* **64**: 1033(2007).

13. Keith S Cinnamon: *Nutrition Today* **43**: 263-266. (2008).

14. Hlebowicz J, Darwiche G, Bjorgell O, Almer LO.. *Am J Clin Nutr* **85**: 1552-1556. (2007).

15. Imparl-Radosevich J, Deas S, Polansky MM, Baedke DA, Ingebritsen TS, Anderson RA, Graves DJ. *Hormone Res* **50:** 177-182. (1998).

16. Cao H, Polansky MM, Anderson RA *Arch Biochem Biophys* **459**: 214-222. (2007).

17. Jarvill-Taylor KJ, Anderson RA, Graves DJ. *J Am Coll Nutr* **20:** 327-336, (2001).

18. Langner E, Greifenberg S, Gruenwald J.. *Adv Ther* **15:** 25-44. (1998).

19. Lamb AB.. *Anaesthesia* **48**: 1118(1993).

20. Srivastava KC, Mustafa T. *Med Hypothesis* **29**: 25-28. (1989).

21. Schulick P. Ginger: common spice or Wonder drug? Herbal Free Press, Brattleboro, Vermont, USA(1993).

22. Reddy AC, Lokesh BR. *Mol Cell Biochem* **111:** 117-124, (1992).

23. Lee YB, Kim YS, Ashmore CR *J Food Science* **51**: 20-23 , (1986).

24. Jagetia GC, Baliga MS, Venkatesh P, Ulloor JN *Radiation Res* **160:** 584-591, (2003).

25. Fuhrman B, Rosenblat M, Hayek T, Coleman R, Aviram M. *J Nutr* **130**: 1124-1131, (2000).

26. Afshari AT, Shirpoor A, Farshid A, Saadatian R, rasmi Y, Saboory E, Llkhanizadeh B, Allameh A. **101**: 148-153, (2007).

27. Masuda Y, Kikuzaki H, Hisamoto M, Nakatani N. *Biofactors* **21**: 293-296,(2008).

28. Zhang F, Altorki NK, Mestre JR. *Carcinogenesis* **20**: 445-451,(1999).

29. Toda S, Miyase T, Arichi H, Tanizawa H, Takino Y L. *Chem Pharm Bull* **33**: 1725-1728, (1985).

30. Selvam R, Subramanian L, Gayathri R, Angayarkanni N *J Ethnopharmacology* **47**: 59-67, (1995).

31. Srinivas L, Shalini VK, Shylaja M. *Arch Biochem Biophys* **292**: 617-623, (1999).

32. Cohly HHP, Asad S, Das SK, Angel MF, Rao M, *Int J Mol Sci:* **4:** 22-33, (2003).

33. US Department of Agriculture. Nutrient database fro standard reference. Release 14. Washington DC: US Department of Agriculture, (2001).

34. Srichamroen A, Thomson ABR, Field CJ, Basu TK *Nutr Res* ,**29**:49-54. (2009).

35. Srichamroen A, Field CJ, Thomson ABR, Basu TK.. *J Clin Biochem Nutr* **43:** 167-174. (2008).

36. Bhaumick D, Acharya A, Basu TK. *World Health J* : **1**: 263-269. (2008).

37. Broca C, Manteghetti M, Gross R, Baissac Y, Jacob M, Petit P, Sauvaire Y, Ribes G. *European J Pharmacol* **390**: 339-345, (2000).

38. Kaviarasan S, Naik GH, Gangabhagirathi R, Anuradha CV, Priyadarsini KI *Food Chemistry* **103**: 31-37, (2007).

39. Kaviarasan S, Anuradha CV. *Pharmazie* **62**: 299-304, (2007).

40. Ravikumar P, Anuradha CV. *Phytotherapy Res* **13:** 197-201, (1999).

41. Dixit P, Ghaskadbi S, Mohan H, Devasagayam TPA. *Phytotherapy res* **19**: 977-983. (2005).

42. Dragland S, Senoo H, Wake K, Holte K, Blomloff R *J Nutr* **133:** 1286-1290. (2003).

43. Lagouri V, Blekas G, Tsimidou M, Kokkini S, Boskou D *Zeitschrift fur Lebensmitteluntersuchung und-Forschung* **197**: 20-23. (1993).

44. Chun S, Vattem DA, Lin Y, Shetty K. *Process Biochem* **40**: 809-816, (2005).

45. Cervato G, Carabelli M, Gervasio S, Cittera A, Cazzola R, Cestaro B *J Food Biochem* **24**: 453-465, (2007).

46. Vekiari SA, Oreopoulou V, Tzia C, Thomopoulos CD. *J Am Oil Chemists Soc* **70**: 483-487. (1993).

47. Lagouri V, Boskou D. Internat *J Food Sci Nutr* **47**: 495-497(1996).

48. Leung AY, Foster S. Encyclopedia of common natural ingredients used in food. In: Drugs and Cosmetics, 2nd edition, John Wiley & Sons, New York. (1996).

49. Julian HR and Simon JE Antioxidant activity of basil. In: Trends in new crops and new uses (eds. Jenick J and Whipkey K), ASHS Press, Alexandra, VA, pp. 575-579. (2002).

50. Simon JE, Quinn J , Murray RG Basil: A source of essential oils. In: Advances in new crops (eds. Janick J and Simon JE), Timber Press, Portland, OR, pp. 484-489. (1990).

51. Phippen WB, Simon JE. *J Hered* **91**: 289-296, (2000).

52. Gulcin I, Elmastas M, Aboul-Enein HW *Phytotherapy res* **21**: 354-361. (2007).

53. Jayasinghe C, Gotoh N, Aoki T. *J Agri Food Chem* **51**: 4442-4449. (2003).

54. Juntachote T, Berghofer E, Bauer F. *Food Chem* **100**: 129-135. (2007).

55. Lee Y, Howard LR, Villalon B. J Food Sci **60**: 473-476. (2006).

56. Sun T, Xu Z, Wu C-T, Janes M, Prinyawiwatkul W, No HK. *J Food Sci* **72:** 98-102(2007).

57. Yoshioka M, St-Pierre S, drapeau V *Br J Nutr* 82: 115-123. (1999).

58. Lejeune MP, Kovacs EM, Westerterp-Plantenga MS. *Br J Nutr* **9:** 651-659. (2003).

59. Ahuja DK, Robertson IK, Geraghty DP, Ball MJ. *Am J Clin Nutr* **84**: 63-69. (2006).

60. Yoshioka M, Imanaga M, Ueyama H, Yamane M, Yoshika K, Boivin A, St-Amand J, Tanaka H, Kiyonaga A.. *Br J Nutr* **91**: 991-995. (2004).

61. Ohnuki K, Haramizu S, Oki K, Watanabe T, Yazawa S, Fushiki T. Biosci *Biotechnol Biochem* **65**: 2735-2740. (2001).

62. Inoue N, Matsunaga Y, Satoh H, Takahashi M. *Biosci Biotechnol Biochem* 71: 380-389. (2007).

63. Kramer RE.. *J Am Oil Chemists Soc* **62:** 111-113. (2007).

64. Lean LP, Mohamed S. *J Sci Food Agric* **79**: 1817-1822. (1999).

65. Srivastava KC and Mustafa T. *Prostaglandins Leukotrienes and Essential Fatty acids* **38:** 255-266. (1989).

66. Schwarz K, Ernst H, Ternes W J *Sci Food Agri* **70**: 217-223 (1999).

67. Bandara MS, Tanino KK, Acharya SN. Research Signpost, Kerala, India. pp. 173-194. (2007).

68. Perry NS, Bollen C, Perry EK, Ballard C. *Pharmacol Biochem Behav* **75:** 651-659. (2003).

69. Madsen HL, Bertelsen G.. *Trends Food Sci Technol* **6**: 271-277. (1995).

70. Ize-Ludlow D, Ragone S, Bernstein JN. *JAMA* **291**: 562-563. (2004).

71. Keawpradub N, Salaeh S, Muangwong S. Songklanakarin *J Sci Technol* **23**: 527-536. (2001).

72. Abu-Amsha R, Croft KD, Puddey IB, Proudfoot JM, Beilin L *J. Clin Sci* **91**: 449-458. (1996).

73. Newall CA, Anderson IA, Philpson JD. Herbal medicine: A guide for healthcare professionals. London, UK, Pharmaceutical Press. (1996).

74. Schwarz K, Ternes W *Zettschbrift fur Lebensmitted-Untersuchung und-Forschung* **195**: 95-98. (1992).

75. Wang JG, Anderson RA, Graham GM, Chu MC, Sauer MV, Guarnaccia MM, Lobo RA. *Fertil Steril* **88**: 240-243. (2007).

76. Spricigo CB, Pinto LT, Bolzan A, Novais AF. *J Supercritical Fluids* **15:** 253-259. (1999).

77. Valderrama JC.. *Phytochemistry* **55:** 505-511. (2000).

78. Kumaravelu P, Subramaniyam S, Dakshinamoorthy DP, Devaraj NS *J Nutr Biochem* 7: 23-28. (1996).

79. Tezuka Y, Irikawa S, Kaneko T *J Ethnopharmacol* 77: 209-217. (2001).

80. Krisnakantha TP, Lokesh BR. Indian *J Biochem Biophys* **30**: 133-134. (1993).

81. Guerra NB, Melo EA, Filho JM *J Food Comp Analysis* **18:** 193-199. (2005).

82. Thippeswamy NB, Naidu KA *Europ Food Res Technol* **220**: 472-476. (2005).

83. Mishra BM, Prakash D Internat *J Food Sci Nutr* **56**: 473-481. (2005).

84. Melo EA, Bion FM, Filho JM, Guerra NB. *Europ J Lipid Sci Technol* **105**: 483-487. (2003).

Spices for Taste and Flavour: Nutraceuticals for Human Health

K. Srinivasan

Spices are traditionally consumed as food adjuncts to enhance sensory quality of foods, and are also used in traditional systems of medicine for ages having been recognized to possess physiological effects beneficial to human health. By providing bioactives, spices significantly contribute to human health and may be considered as the first ever functional food. By making foods palatable without salt and fat, spices assist in reduced daily intake of sodium and meeting healthy fat intake. In recent decades, many health beneficial attributes of these common food adjuncts have been experimentally documented from numerous animal studies and clinical trials. The antioxidant and hypocholesterolemic properties of spices have far-reaching nutraceutical value. The antioxidant properties of bioactive compounds present in spices are of particular interest in view of the impact of suppression of oxidative stress in the development of degenerative diseases such as cardiovascular disease, neurodegenerative disease, inflammatory disease and cancer. Spices thus deserve to be considered as the natural and necessary component of our daily nutrition, beyond their role in imparting taste and flavour to our food.

Introduction

Spices are traditionally consumed as food adjuncts to enhance sensory quality of foods, the quantity and variety consumed in tropical countries being particularly extensive. Besides contributing to flavour, colour and aroma to our everyday diet, spices have also been long recognized to possess physiological effects supposed to be beneficial to human health. They act as stimulus to the digestive system, relieve digestive disorders, and some spices are of antiseptic value. Their attributes such as tonic, carminative, stomachic, diuretic, and anti-spasmodic ? largely empirical nevertheless efficacious, have found pharmacological applications in the indigenous systems of medicine. With the long history of the use of spices dating back to 5000 years BC, and spices significantly contributing to human health by providing bioactives, these may be considered as the first ever recorded functional foods. Spices make foods palatable without salt and hence assist in the desirable reduced daily intake of sodium. Similarly, they make foods palatable without fat, thus enabling to meet healthy fat intake. The use of spices also encourages variety in food intake, thus supporting nutrient diversity by encouraging number of food choices. They have captured the attention of scientific community in recent times as potential providers of health benefits.

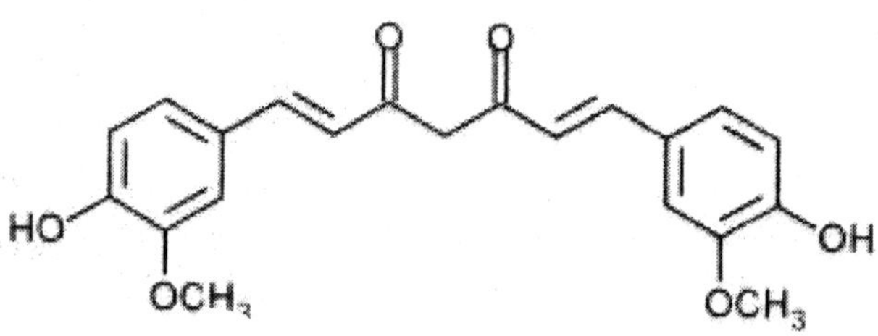

Curcumin (*Curcuma longa*)

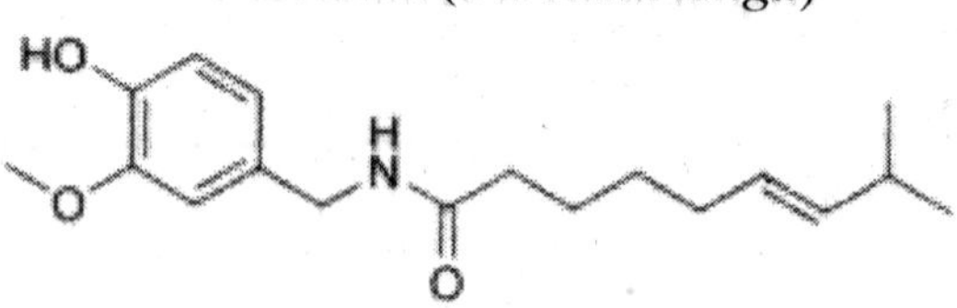

Capsaicin (*Capsicum annuum*)

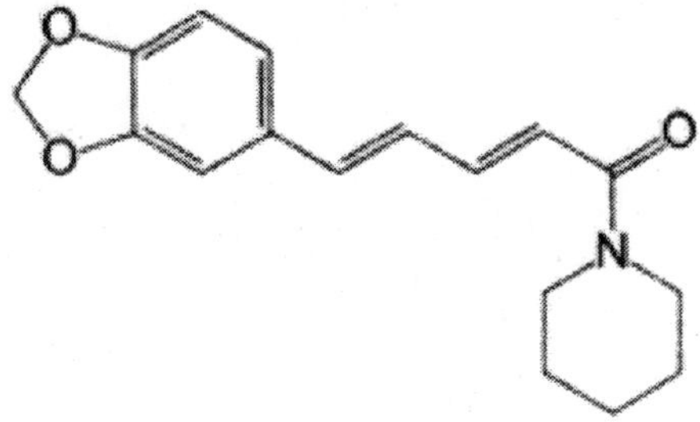

Piperine (*Piper nigrum*)

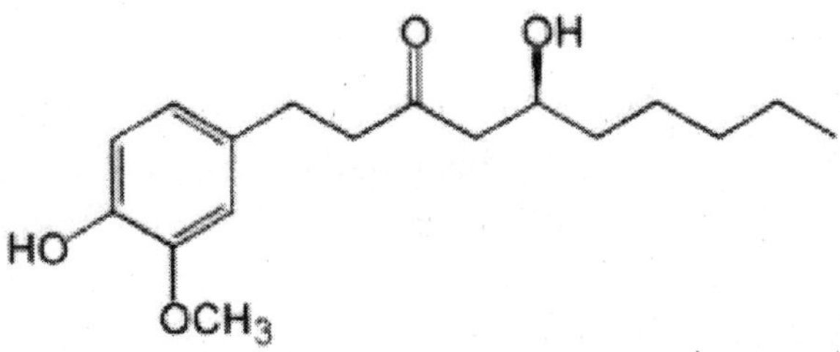

Gingerol (*Zinger officinale*)

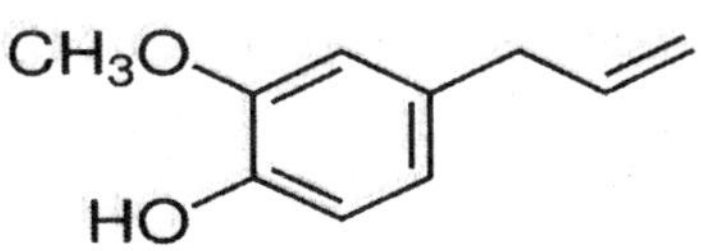

Eugenol (*Eugenia caryophyllus*)

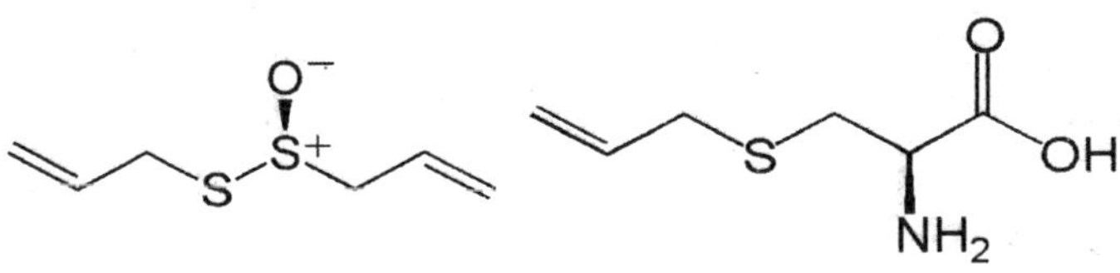

Allicin and S-allyl cysteine (*Allium sativa*)

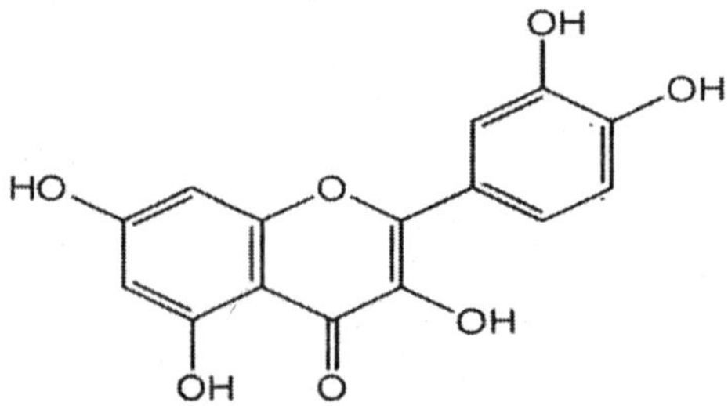

Quercetin (*Allium cepa*)

Fig.1. Structure of spice bioactive compounds

Nutraceutical attributes of spices

Spices do not contribute anything significant to human nutrition, while they are valued as flavour modifiers to make food palatable. Interestingly, the protein content in spices varies from 4.5 % in rosemary leaves to 31.5% in mustard, fat level varies from 0.6 % in garlic to 42.6 % in mustard. The mineral content ranges from 2.3 % in marjoram to 16.7% in basil leaves. While some of them contain significant levels of vitamins and minerals, a few spices are also rich sources of dietary fibre. Amongst common spices consumed, the dietary fibre is highest in chilli, as high as 43.3% while black pepper (27.8%), coriander (36.2%), cumin (23.0%), fennel (28.7%) and fenugreek (33.5%) also are rich sources of dietary fibre, both soluble as well as insoluble. However, due to low levels of consumption of spices, their impact on nutrient makeup may not be as dramatic as other food ingredients.

In the last 3 decades, several health beneficial effects of spices have been experimentally documented which suggest that the use of these food adjuncts extends beyond taste and flavour.[1] The emerging research literature suggests that specific spices may confer unique health benefits. Although human studies are limited, considerable attention to this has been drawn because of the positive results from *in vitro* and *in vivo* animal studies.

Digestive stimulant action

The digestive stimulant action of spices is probably the most common experience. Several spices such as ginger, mint, ajowan, cumin, fennel, coriander and garlic are common remedies used in traditional medicines or ingredients of pharmacological preparations to cure digestive disorders. The mechanism of digestive stimulant action of spices has been recently understood by extensive animal studies.[2] It has been evidenced that many commonly consumed spices (curcumin, capsaicin, ginger, fenugreek, mustard, cumin, coriander, ajowan, tamarind and onion) stimulate bile acid production by the liver and its secretion into bile.[3,4] Bile acids play a major role in fat digestion and absorption. Several spices are also evidenced to stimulate the activity of digestive enzymes of pancreas, particularly lipase and terminal digestive enzymes of small intestinal mucosa.[5,6] As a result of increased digestive capability, the spice fed animals showed a reduced food transit time.[7]

Antidiabetic potential

Among spices that have been evaluated for antidiabetic attribute, fenugreek seeds, garlic and onion, and their sulfur compounds, turmeric and its yellow principle, curcumin have been found to be effective in improving the glycemic status and glucose tolerance in diabetic animals / type-2 diabetic patients.[8] Animal studies and clinical trials on antidiabetic properties of fenugreek and onion have been particularly extensive, while human studics arc limitcd in the case of garlic and turmeric. Studies have unequivocally demonstrated the antidiabetic potential of fenugreek in both type-1 and type-2 diabetes. Addition of fenugreek seeds to the diets of diabetic patients or animals results in a fall in blood glucose and improvement in glucose tolerance.[9-10] The hypoglycemic effect is attributed to the fibre and gum, which constitute as much as 52% of the seeds. The fibre-rich fenugreek is believed to delay gastric emptying by direct interference with glucose absorption.

Garlic and onion are two other spices, which have been widely tested for their antidiabetic potential. Both these spices have been shown to be hypoglycemic in different diabetic animal models and in limited human trials[8]. The hypoglycemic potency of garlic and onion is attributed to the disulfide compounds present in them, di(2-propenyl) disulfide and 2-propenylpropyl disulfide respectively, which cause direct or indirect stimulation of insulin secretion by the pancreas.[11,12] In addition, they may also have insulin-sparing action by protecting from sulfhydryl inactivation by reacting with endogenous thiol-containing molecules such as cysteine, glutathione, and serum albumins. Nephropathy is a common complication in chronic diabetes.

Turmeric is another spice claimed to possess beneficial hypoglycemic effect and to improve glucose tolerance in a limited number of studies. Nephropathy is a common complication in chronic diabetes. High blood cholesterol is an added risk factor that determines the rate of decline of kidney function in diabetic situation. Dietary curcumin (of turmeric) and onion have been found to have a promising ameliorating influence on the severity of renal lesions in streptozotocin diabetic rats.[13,14] Hypocholesterolemic effect of these spices as well as the ability to lower lipid peroxidation under diabetic condition is implicated in the amelioration of renal lesions. Capsaicin of red chilli has been shown to be useful in diabetic neuropathy; in a study involving 219 patients, topical application of 0.075% capsaicin cream was effective in pain management.[15] These antidiabetic spices may be used in conjunction with anti-diabetic drugs to have better therapeutic potential and to minimize drug dosage.

Anti-atherogenic and Cardioprotective effect

a) Hypolipidemic influence

Several common spices have been evaluated for cholesterol lowering effect in a variety of experimental situations in both animals and humans and these studies have been reviewed recently.[16]

Garlic, onion, fenugreek, turmeric and red pepper are found to be effective as hypocholesterolemic agents under various conditions of experimentally induced hyper-cholesterolemia / hyperlipidemia. Garlic, Fenugreek, and onion are effective in humans with hyperlipidemic condition.

Consumption of garlic or garlic oil has been associated with a reduction in total cholesterol, low-density lipoprotein cholesterol, and triglyceride levels. There are more than 25 clinical research concerning garlic and its preparations.[17] With the introduction of dehydrated garlic powder containing a standardized level of the parent sulfur compound - alliin, effective clinical work could be undertaken with a relatively low and acceptable daily dosage of 300 - 900 mg (equivalent to 1 clove of garlic). Many clinical studies have indicated that consuming one clove of garlic (or equivalent) daily will have at least 10% cholesterol-lowering effect.[18] A modest 0.41 mmol/L decrease in serum cholesterol has been evidenced in 780 patients taking 600-900 mg standardized garlic extract per day as supplement.[19] Dietary supplementation with aged garlic extract showed better beneficial effects relative to fresh garlic, on the lipid profile and blood pressure of moderately hypercholesterolemic subjects.[16] While garlic supplementation significantly decreased both total and LDL cholesterol in hypercholesterolemic subjects, co-administration of garlic with fish oil had a better beneficial effect on serum lipid and lipoprotein concentrations by providing a combined lowering of total cholesterol, LDL cholesterol and triglyceride concentration as well as the ratios of total cholesterol to HDL cholesterol and LDL cholesterol to HDL cholesterol.[16]

Fenugreek seeds were hypocholesterolemic in rats with hyperlipidemia induced by either high fat or a high cholesterol diet.[16] Defatted fenugreek seed was effective in diabetic hyper-cholesterolemia in dogs and in humans. The hypolipidemic effectiveness of turmeric / curcumin,[20] red pepper/ capsaicin[21,22] and of onion and garlic[23,24] has been periodically reviewed. Spice compounds ? curcumin and capsaicin have been associated with a decrease in LDL cholesterol and an increase in HDL cholesterol levels in animal studies.

b) Anti-thrombotic property

Besides the beneficial effect on serum lipid profile (Lowering of LDL cholesterol and triglyceride levels), the anti-platelet aggregation and the anti-platelet adhesion properties of several spices also contribute to cardiovascular protection. The spices / spice compounds documented to have inhibitory effect on platelet aggregation are: garlic, onion, curcumin, cuminaldehyde, eugenol, and zingerone. Garlic in particular exhibits anti-thrombotic and hypotensive properties, both of which also contribute to cardiovascular protection besides the hypolipidemic properties. Aged garlic extract has been associated with anti-clotting, as well as modest reductions in blood pressure. The anti-platelet aggregation, the anti-platelet adhesion and the anti-proliferation properties of aged garlic extracts appear to contribute more to the cardiovascular protection than the hypolipidemic properties.

c) Suppression of LDL oxidation

Antioxidant properties of spices are of particular interest in view of the impact of oxidative modification of LDL-cholesterol in the development of atherosclerosis. In recent years, a substantial body of evidence has indicated that free radicals contribute to cardiovascular disease. Oxidative modification of LDL is hypothesized to play a key role during the development of atherosclerosis. Since spices have high antioxidant concentrations that have the potential to inhibit the oxidation of LDL, the use of antioxidant spices is a promising proposition.

d) Thermogenic influence

Obesity related insulin resistance has emerged as a potent risk factor for cardiovascular disease. Dietary factors that affect satiety and thermogenesis could play an important role in determining the prevalence and severity of this problem. Among spices that may have a role to play in this regard, red pepper (or its pungent principle capsaicin)[25] and garlic are promising and more data are required to substantiate the benefit. The use of spices to displace fats and salt in the diet may reduce cardiovascular risk.

Anti-lithogenic effect

Persistent lithogenic diet leads to cholesterol saturation in bile resulting in formation of cholesterol crystals, i.e., gallstones in gall bladder. Studies on experimental induction of cholesterol gallstones in mice and hamsters by feeding a lithogenic diet have revealed that the incidence of gallstones is 40-50% lower when the animals are maintained on 0.5% curcumin or 0.015% capsaicin containing diets.[26] Animal studies have also revealed significant regression of preformed cholesterol gallstones by these spice principles in a 10-week feeding trial.[27] The antilithogenic potential of other known hypocholesterolemic spices – garlic, onion and fenugreek seeds have also been recently evidenced in animal studies.[28,29] The anti-lithogenicity of these spices is attributable to the lowering of cholesterol concentration and enhancing the bile acid concentration, both of which contribute to lowering of cholesterol saturation index and hence its crystallization. In addition to their ability to lower cholesterol saturation index, the antilithogenecity of these spice principles may also be due to their influence on biliary proteins.[30]

Anti-inflammatory property

With increasing interest in alternatives to non-steroidal anti-inflammatory agents in the management of chronic inflammation, the use of food based approaches is emerging. Lipid peroxides play a crucial role in arthritis and other inflammatory diseases. Turmeric happens to be the earliest anti-inflammatory drug known in the indigenous system of medicine in India. Turmeric extract, curcuminoids, and volatile oil of turmeric have been found to be effective as anti-inflammatory in several studies involving mice, rats, rabbits, and pigeons. The efficacy of curcuminoids was also established in carrageenan induced foot paw edema in mice and rats and in cotton pellet granuloma pouch tests in rats[20]. Curcumin was considered to be advantageous over aspirin because it selectively inhibits the synthesis of the anti-inflammatory prostaglandin T_xA_2, without affecting the synthesis of prostacyclin (PgI_2) which is an important factor preventing vascular thrombosis.[31] Both *in vitro* and *in vivo* animal studies have documented the anti-inflammatory potential of spice principles curcumin (of turmeric), capsaicin (of red pepper) and eugenol (of clove). Animal studies have revealed that curcumin and capsaicin also lower the incidence and severity of arthritis and also delay the onset of adjuvant induced arthritis. These spice principles also inhibited the formation of arachidonate metabolites (PgE_2, leukotrienes).

Anti-inflammatory effect of curcumin (400 mg) in patients undergone surgery for hernia / hydrocele was found comparable to that of phenylbutazone (100 mg) (Satoskar *et al*, 1986). In rheumatoid arthritis patients, administration of curcumin (1.2 g/day) produced significant improvement similar to phenylbutazone.[32] Recently, capsaicin has received considerable attention as a pain reliever. In two trials with 70 and 21 patients with osteoarthritis and rheumatoid arthritis, topical application of creams containing 0.025% or 0.075% capsaicin was an effective and safe alternative to analgesics employed in systemic medications which are often associated with potential side effects.[33] Capsaicin has also been suggested for the initial management of neuralgia consequent to herpes infection. There is also evidence for the benefit of ginger in ameliorating arthritic knee pain, although the effectiveness is lesser than that of ibuprofen. Ginger doses of 0.5 - 1.0 g per day were efficacious in osteoarthritis and rheumatoid arthritis. Experimental studies have shown that ginger constituents inhibit arachidonic acid metabolism which is involved in the inflammation process (a key pathway in inflammation).

Natural anti-inflammatory compounds of spices (curcumin, capsaicin, gingerol) appear to operate by inhibiting one or more of the steps linking pro-inflammatory stimuli with COX activation, such as the blocking by curcumin of NFkB translocation into the nucleus. It has been shown recently that the natural anti-inflammatory compounds such curcumin were as effective as indomethacin (a non-steroidal anti-inflammatory drug) in inhibiting aberrant crypt foci in the rat.

Antimutagenicity and anti-cancer effect

Recently, considerable attention has been focused on identifying naturally occurring chemopreventive substances capable of inhibiting, retarding, or reversing the multi-stage carcinogenesis. Phenolic substances present in spices have been reported to possess substantial anticarcinogenic activities. The majority of these naturally occurring phenolics possess antioxidative and anti-inflammatory properties, which appear to contribute to their chemo-preventive or chemoprotective activity.[22]

There are a number of *in vitro* studies and rodent *in vivo* studies suggesting that spices may have a chemopreventive effect against the early initiating stages of cancer. As yet, there are no data indicating that spices have an anticarcinogenic effect in humans. Spices may act through several mechanisms to provide protection against cancer. Certain phytochemicals from spices have been shown to inhibit one or more of the stages of the cancer process (initiation, promotion, growth and metastasis). Inhibition of phase I metabolic enzymes (involved in procarcinogen activation) and induction of phase II metabolic enzymes (involved in carcinogen dcactivation) may account for the chemopreventive effects of spices. Spices may also protect against oxidative stress and inflammation, both of which are a risk factor for cancer initiation and promotion (as well as other pathological conditions). Spices contain several natural antioxidant biomolecules lipid-soluble that may protect against the generation of genotoxic lipid peroxidation peroxides.

Spices that have antioxidant property can function as antimutagens. Since, mutagenesis has a direct bearing on cancer initiation, anti-mutagenic spices can probably be anticarcinogenic too. Turmeric / curcumin, garlic / its sulfur compounds have been shown to be antimutagenic in several experimental systems. *In vivo* studies in experimental animals suggest that turmeric and curcumin inhibit the formation of mutagens. Mice and rats maintained on turmeric or curcumin-containing diet excreted lower levels of mutagenic metabolites as well as carcinogens than the controls.[34,35] Turmeric and curcumin also inhibited the mutagenicity of cigarette and beedi smoke condensates as also that of a tobacco-based dentifrice and curcumin was found to inhibit nitrosation of methylurea *in vitro*.[36,37] Studies on smokers revealed that administration of curcumin (1.5 g / day) for 30 days resulted in a significant reduction in the urinary excretion of mutagens.[38] Eugenol (the flavour constituent of cloves) and mustard seeds (that contain dithiolthione) also produce anti-mutagenic effect by protecting the cell from damage to DNA. Dithiolthiones are documented to have protective effect against liver toxicity induced by some chemicals and the fungal toxin aflatoxin.

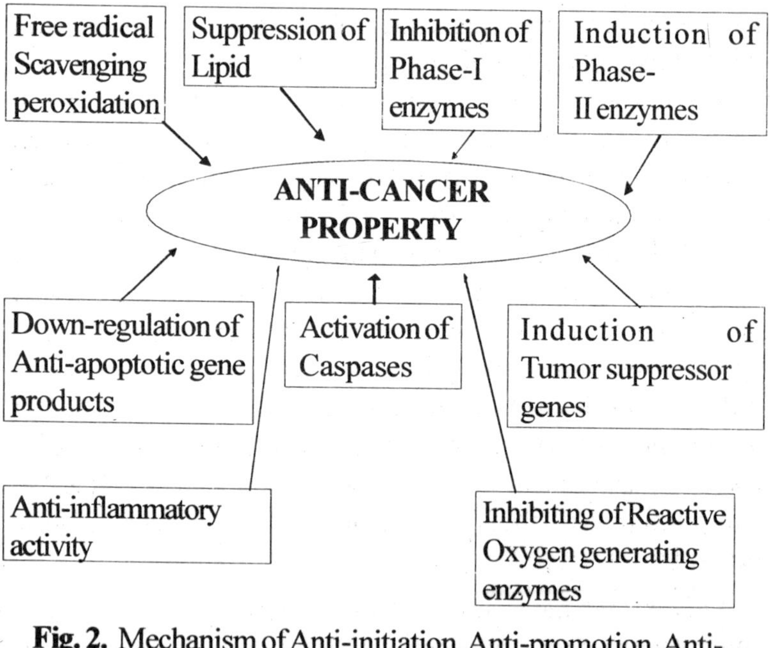

Fig. 2. Mechanism of Anti-initiation, Anti-promotion, Anti-progression and Anti-metastasis potential of spices

Spices (or their extracts / constituents) with known anticarcinogenic effects in animal models of cancer include turmeric, garlic and ginger. Turmeric has been found to have chemopreventive effects against cancers of the skin, forestomach, liver, colon, and oral cancer in mice. The anticancer potential of curcumin as evidenced by both preclinical and clinical studies has been exhaustively reviewed recently.[39] Animal studies involving experimental induction of tumour of specific tissues with potent carcinogens (such as benz(a-)pyrene, 7,12-dimethylbenzanthracene, 3-methylcholanthrene, 12-*O*-tetradecanoylphorbol-13-acetate, 1,2-dimethylhydrazine, etc.) have revealed significant reduction of the incidence of tumour in curcumin treatment. Several studies indicate that curcumin can suppress both tumour initiation and tumour promotion. Some of these studies, especially studies of skin tumorigenesis have also employed topical application of curcumin.[39] It has been shown that the inhibition of arachidonic acid metabolism, modulation of cellular signal transduction pathways, inhibition of hormone, growth factor, and oncogene activity are some of the mechanisms by which curcumin causes tumour suppression. Chemopreventive activity of curcumin is observed when administered prior to, during, and after carcinogen treatment as well as when it is given only during promotion / progression phase of colon carcinogenesis in rats. Curcumin is a powerful inhibitor of the proliferation of several tumour cells. With many evidences suggesting that curcumin can suppress tumour initiation, promotion and metastasis, and with proven safety of its consumption (up to 10 g per day), curcumin offers enormous potential in the prevention and therapy of cancer[39].

Cancer preventive ability of garlic has been indicated by etiological studies wherein higher intake of Allium products is associated with reduced risk of several types of cancers, especially stomach and colorectal.[40] Garlic is effective in the detoxification of carcinogens through its effects on phase I and phase II enzymes. Diallyl disulfide of garlic is an efficient inhibitor of the phase I enzyme cytochrome P-450 and significantly enhances a variety of phase

II enzymes including GSH-transferase, quinone reductase and UDP-glucuronyl transferase, which are responsible for the detoxification of carcinogens. Several mechanisms have been proposed to explain the cancer-preventive effects of garlic and its organosulfur compounds, as has been recently reviewed[4.1] These include inhibition of mutagenesis, modulation of enzyme activities thus suppressing bioactivation of carcinogen molecules, inhibition of carcinogen-DNA adduct formation, free radical scavenging, inhibitory effects on cell proliferation and tumor growth, and induction of apoptosis.

Pungent vanilloids especially [6]-gingerol present in ginger (*Zingiber officinale*) have been found to possess potential chemopreventive activities. Prior topical application of [6]-gingerol significantly suppressed the tumor promoter (phorbol ester) stimulated skin inflammation initiated by 7,12-dimethylbenz [a] anthracene in mice.[42] Reactive nitrogen species (RNS), such as nitric oxide (NO) have been proposed as being able to influence signal transduction and cause DNA damage, contributing to carcinogenic processes. [6]-gingerol, a pungent phenolic compound present in ginger is evidenced to be a potent inhibitor of NO synthesis and also an effective protector against peroxynitrite-mediated damage in macrophages.[43] Dietary ginger constituents, galanals A and B, are potent apoptosis inducers in Human T lymphoma cells.

Antioxidant activity

Generation of reactive oxygen species and other free radicals during metabolism is a normal process that is ideally compensated for by an elaborate endogenous antioxidant defense system. Excessive free radicals generation over-balancing the rate of their removal leads to oxidative stress. Oxidative damage has been implicated in the etiology of disease processes such as cardiovascular disease, inflammatory diseases, cancer, neurodegenerative diseases, and other degenerative diseases. Antioxidants are compounds that hinder the oxidative processes and thereby delay or suppress oxidative stress. The bioactive compounds present in spices which possess potent anti-atherogenic, anti-inflammatory, anti-mutagenic and cancer preventive activities are in fact antioxidants that are experimentally evidenced to control cellular oxidative stress and thereby exert a beneficial role in preventing oxidative stress mediated diseases.

Most of the health effects of spices on cancer, cardiovascular disease, inflammatory diseases and neurodegenerative diseases may be mediated through their potent antioxidant effects. The antioxidant properties of spices are of particular interest in view of the impact of oxidative modifications of LDL-cholesterol in the development of atherosclerosis. Supression of oxidative stress and inflammation by spices is important in their cancer preventive role, since both oxidative stress and inflammation are a risk factor for cancer initiation and promotion. The antioxidative effects of curcumin, eugenol, capsaicin, piperine, gingerol, garlic, onion, and fenugreek have been experimentally evidenced.[44] The studies to this effect are exhaustive and experimental evidences are plenty in the case of curcumin of turmeric and eugenol of clove. Studies with several *in vitro* systems as well as *in vivo* animal studies have revealed that spice principles curcumin, eugenol and capsaicin have beneficial antioxidant property by quenching oxygen free radicals, by inhibiting the production of reactive oxygen radicals, and by enhancing the antioxidant enzyme activities.

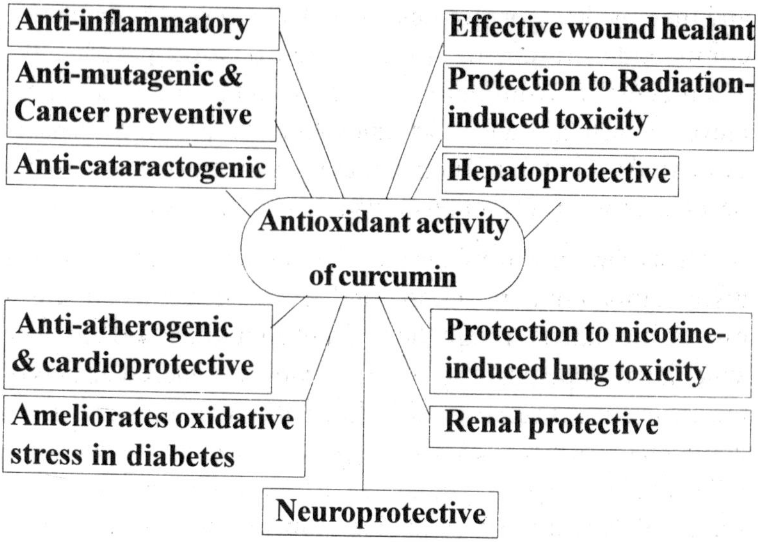

Fig. 3. Health implications of antioxidant property

The antioxidant activity of the spice compounds in mammalian system involve one or more of the following: (1) free radical scavenging, (2) suppressing of lipid peroxidation, (3) enhancing the antioxidant molecules in tissues, (4) stimulating the activities of endogenous antioxidant enzymes, (5) Inhibition of the activity of inducible nitric oxide synthase, (6) Inhibition of LDL oxidation, (6) Inhibition of enzymes of arachidonate metabolism - 5-lipoxygenase and 2-cyclooxygenase enzymes. By virtue of antioxidant activity, curcumin has been documented to be anti-inflammatory, anti-mutagenic and cancer preventive, anti-atherogenic and cardioprotective, hepatoprotective, neuroprotective, anti-cataractogenic, effective wound healant, etc.

Conclusions

By making the food attractive and palatable through flavour, aroma and colour, spices can reduce the need to use less healthy ingredients such as salt, fat or sugar. Many health beneficial attributes of these common food adjuncts have been experimentally evidenced in the past few decades which include: digestive stimulant action, anti-atherogenic and cardioprotective potential,

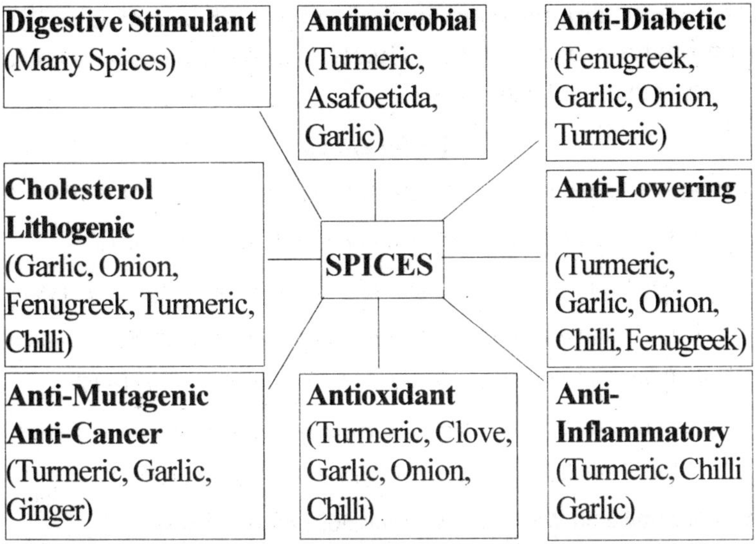

Fig.4. Summary of multiple health effects of spices

antilithogenic property, antidiabetic influence, Anti-inflammatory property, and cancer preventive potential. The antioxidant and hypolipidemic properties of spices have far-reaching nutraceutical value. The antioxidant properties of bioactive compounds present in spices are of particular interest in view of the impact of suppression of oxidative stress in the development of degenerative diseases such as cardiovascular disease, neurodegenerative disease, inflammatory disease and cancer. Spices thus deserve to be considered as the natural and necessary component of our daily nutrition, beyond their role in imparting taste and flavour to our food. It is presumed that the additive and synergistic effects of the complex mixture of phytochemicals present in vegetables, fruits, herbs and spices are largely responsible for the health effects offered by Indian and Mediterranean diets which are generally associated with lower incidence rates of some of the chronic diseases of ageing including cardiovascular disease and certain forms of cancer. The liberal consumption of spices is proved to be safe to derive their beneficial effects. Since each of the spices possesses more than one health beneficial property and that there is also a possibility of synergy among them in their action when consumed in combination, a spiced diet is likely to make life not only more 'spicy' but more healthy also.

References

1. K.Srinivasan. *Food Rev.Int.* **21**, 167-188 (2005).

2. K.Platel and K.Srinivasan. *J.Med.Res.* **119**, 167-179 (2004).

3. K.Sambaiah and K.Srinivasan. *J.Food Sci.Technol.* **28**, 35-38 (1991).

4. K.Platel and K.Srinivasan. *Nutr.Res.* **20**, 1493-1503 (2000).

5. K.Platel and Srinivasan. *Int.J.Food Sci.Nutr.* **47**, 55-59 (1996).

6. K.Platel and K.Srinivasan.. *Nahrung,* **44**, 42-46 (2000).

7. K.Platel and K.Srinivasan.. *Nutr.Res.* **21**, 1309-1314 (2001).

8. K.Srinivasan. *Int.J.Food Sci.Nutr.* **56**, 399-414 (2005).

9. R.D.Sharma. *Nutr.Res.* **6**, 1353-1364 (1986).

10. R.D.Sharma, A.Sarkar and D.K.Hazra. *Nutr.Res.* **16**, 1331-1339 (1996).

11. Kumudkumari, B.C.Mathew BC and K.T.Augusti. *Indian J.Biochem.Biophys.* **32**, 49-54 (1995).

12. K.T.Augusti and C.G.Sheela. *Experientia,* **52**, 115-119 (1996).

13. P.S.Babu and K.Srinivasan. *Mol.Cell.Biochem.* **181**, 87-96 (1998).

14. P.S.Babu and K.Srinivasan.. *J.Nutr.Biochem.* **10**, 477-483 (1999).

15. The Capsaicin Study Group. *Diabetic Care,* **15**,159-165 (1992).

16. K.Srinivasan, K.Sambaiah and N.Chandrasekhara. *Food Rev.Int.* **20**, 187-220 (2004).

17. J.Kleijnen, P.Knipschild and G.Terriet. **28**, 535-544 (1989).

18. J.M.Gore and J.E.Dalen. *JAMA*, **271**, 1660-1661 (1994).

19. C.Stevinson, M.H.Pittler and E.Ernst. *Ann.Intern.Med.* **133**, 420-429 (2000).

20. R.C.Srimal. *Fitoterapia,* LXVIII, 483-490 (1997).

21. T.Suzuki and K.Iwai. Constituents of red pepper species: Chemistry, biochemistry, pharmacology and food science of the pungent principle of *Capsicum* species. In: Brossi, A., ed. *The Alkaloids – Chemistry & Pharmacology*; Vol. 23, New York: Academic Press, 227-299 (1984).

22. Y.J.Surh. *Food Chem.Toxicol.* **40**, 1091-1097 (2002).

23. J.F.Carson. *Food Rev.Int.* **3**, 71-103 (1987).

24. M.K.Jain and R.Apitz-Castro. Garlic: A matter for heart. In: Charalambouis, G., ed. *Spices, Herbs and edible Fungi.* USA: Elsevier, 311-364 (1994).

25. T.Kawada, K.Hagihara and K.Iwai. *J.Nutr.* **116**, 1272-1278 (1986).

26. M.S.Hussain and N.Chandrasekhara. *Nutr.Res.*, **13**, 349-357 (1993).

27. M.S.Hussain and N.Chandrasekhara. *Nutr.Res.*, **14**, 1561-1574 (1994).

28. S.Vidyashankar, K.Sambaiah and K.Srinivasan.. *Br.J.Nutr.*, doi: 10.1017/S0007114508118748 (2008)

29. R.L.R.Reddy and K.Srinivasan. *Can.J.Physiol. Pharmacol.*, In Press (2009).

30. M.S.Hussain and N.Chandrasekhara. *Indian J. Biochem.Biophys.*, **31**, 407-412 (1994).

31. V.Srivastava. *Arznei Forch.*, **36**, 715-717 (1986).

32. S.D.Deodhar, R.Sethi and R.C.Srimal. *Indian J.Med.Res.* **71**, 632-634 (1980).

33. C.L.Deal.. *Clin.Therap.* **13**, 383-395 (1991).

34. K.Usha. *J.Am.Col.Nutr.* **13**, 519-521 (1994).

35. K.Polasa, B.Sesikaran, T.P.Krishna and K.Krishnaswamy. *Food Chem.Toxicol.* **29**, 699-706 (1991).

36. M.Nagabushan, A.J.Amonkar and S.V.Bhide.. *Food Chem.Toxicol.* **25**, 545-547 (1987).

37. M.Nagabushan, U.J.Nair, A.J.Amonkar, A.V.D'Souza and S.V.Bhide.. *Mutation Res.* **202**, 163-169 (1988).

38. K.Polasa, T.C.Raghuram, T.P.Krishna and K.Krishnaswamy.. *Mutagenesis*, 7, 107-109 (1992).

39. B.B.Aggarwal, A.Kumar and A.C.Bharti.. *Anticancer Res.*, **23**, 363-398 (2003).

40. A.T.Fleischauer and L.Arab. *J Nutr.* **131**, 1032S-40S (2001).

41. A.Sengupta, S.Ghosh and S.Bhattacharjee.. *Asia Pac.J.Cancer Prev.* **5**, 237-245 (2004).

42. Y.J. Surh, K.K. Park, K.S. Chun, L.J. Lee, E. Lee and S.S. Lee. *J.Environ.Pathol. Toxicol.Oncol.* **18**,131-139 (1999).

43. K. Ippoushi, K. Azuma, H. Ito, H. Horie and H. Higashio. *Life Sci.* **73**, 3427-3437 (2003).

44. K.Srinivasan. *Crit.Rev.Food Sci. Nutr.*, In Press (2009).

"Spicing Up" of the Cardiovascular System

Asim K. Duttaroy

Certain plants and spices containing flavonoids have been used for thousands of years in traditional Eastern medicine. A large body of evidence supports that dietary intake of spices may be able to exert some beneficial cardiovascular effects and thereby reduce the risk for cardiovascular morbidity and mortality. Spices are likely to protect cardiovascular system via several mechanisms such as lowering of LDL cholesterol levels, inhibition of ROS and platelet aggregation. The available data are few, and a wide range of dose and type of spices tested making difficult to conclude the beneficial effects of spices on CVD. Long-term clinical trials are needed to definitively clarify the benefits deriving from long-term consumption of spice-rich foods, particularly focussing on the lowest effective levels as well as synergism or antagonistic actions between different classes of flavonoids commonly found in spices.

Introduction

Cardiovascular disease (CVD) includes all diseases that affect the heart and blood vessels, such as coronary heart disease (CHD), coronary artery disease, dyslipidemia, and hypertension. Atherosclerosis, the most common cause of CHD, is the progressive thickening and hardening of the walls of medium-sized and large arteries as a result of inflammation and fat deposits on their inner lining.[1,2] The last decade of evidence has revealed the central role of inflammation in all phases of the atherosclerotic process. Oxidized LDL (oxLDL) exerts a multitude of potentially atherogenic effects in vivo and in vitro.[3] Platelets are also involved in inûammation, atherogenesis and atherothrombosis through the ability to adhere to injured vessels, to accumulate at sites of vascular injury and to release bioactive mediators monolayer formed on the injured vessels provides a surface for leukocyte adhesion and migration.[4,5] Figure 1 shows the obesity/diabetes affecting platelet function. Therefore, hyperactivity of platelets, and their adhesion and aggregation at the site of injury in atherosclerotic vessel walls, is also critically important in the pathogenesis of CVD.[4,5] Platelet reactivity may be increased by production of reactive oxygen species (ROS) as a consequence of oxidative stress; reduction of endothelial antithrombotic properties, and increased availability of proinflammatory mediators, such as chemokines.[6-8] Since oxidative modification of LDL results from lipid peroxidation, both water and lipid soluble antioxidants have been demonstrated in preventing oxidative modification of LDL.[9] In fact the beneficial effects of fruits, vegetables and spices on the cardiovascular system may be explained by the antioxidants content that inhibit the oxidation of membrane lipids, proteins and LDL.[10,11] Recent data however suggesting that the non-antioxidant properties of fruits and vegetables play important roles in preventing diseases.[12,13]

Research on human nutrition has led to an awareness of the health benefits of diet associated non-nutrient components. Specifically, it has been recognized that complex array of naturally occurring bioactive non-nutrients may confer significant long-term health benefits. Spices are food additives used mainly to impart color and flavor and also for other special properties like stimulation of appetite, carminative action and preservation of food.[14] Turmeric, garlic, onion, pepper and cloves are some of the most commonly used spices in culinary preparations.[14] These spices contain phenolic compounds including flavonoids and non-flavonoids and exhibit antioxidant and anti-platelet properties. The active principles of spices such as curcumin (turmeric), quercetin (onion, garlic), capsaicin (capsicum), piperine (pepper), eugenol (cloves) and allyl sulfide (garlic), and herbs have protective effect on the cardiovascular system.[15,16] This article reviews the beneficial effects of spices on the cardiovascular system.

Spices and the Cardiovascular System

Several spices have long been recognized to possess medicinal properties such as tonic, carminative, stomachic antispasmodic, and anti-helminthic. Spices have a diverse array of natural phytochemicals that have complementary and overlapping actions, including antioxidant effects, modulation of detoxification enzymes, stimulation of immune system, reduction of inflammatory responses.[15-19]

Atherosclerosis and Spices

Common conditions predisposing to atherosclerosis, such as hypercholesterolemia, hypertension, diabetes, and smoking, are associated with endothelial dysfunction. A common mechanism underlying endothelial dysfunction relates to increased vascular production of reactive oxygen species (ROS). Elevated levels of oxLDL are considered to be one of the major risk factors for atherosclerosis and cardiovascular morbidity. OxLDL has been detected in atherosclerotic lesions and is thought to play a major role in the initiation and progression of atherosclerosis. The early stages of the atherosclerotic process are initiated by accumulation of oxLDL and activation of endothelial cells with subsequent expression of adhesion molecules and increased binding of monocytes to the vascular endothelium. Pro-inflammatory cytokines, such as IL-1 and TNF-α, which are released when endothelial cells are exposed to oxLDL, up-regulate the expression of cell adhesion molecules.[19] Many antioxidants have been found in spices and herbs, and some of them are well known as strong scavengers of active oxygen radicals. Most of the spice phenolic antioxidants are good scavengers of lipid hydroxy radicals, the radical quenching ability of spice active principles could be responsible for the inhibition of oxidation of LDL. Among the spice active principles tested curcumin was the most potent inhibitor at both initiation and propogation phases of oxidation of LDL. Curcumin (diferuloylmethane), a polyphenol, is an active principle of the perennial herb Curcuma longa (commonly known as Turmeric). The yellow-pigmented fraction of turmeric contains curcuminoids, which are chemically related to its principal ingredient, curcumin. The major curcuminoids present in turmeric are demethoxycurcumin (curcumin II), bisdemethoxycurcumin (curcumin III), and the recently identified cyclocurcumin. The major components of commercial curcumin are curcumin I (77%), curcumin II (17%), and curcumin III (3%). The active principles which constitute about 1–4% of raw spices thus impart beneficial properties as natural, dietary antioxidants on oxidation of human LDL. Among the spice principles tested curcumin and capsaicin exhibited significant inhibition at initiation and propagation phases of LDL oxidation, while quercetin was effective during initiation phase only. Daily administration of curcumin (500 mg) for 7 days led to a significant 33% decrease in serum lipid peroxides, a 29% increase in serum HDL cholesterol, and a nearly 12% decrease in total serum cholesterol.[20] Together, these striking findings suggest a potential chemopreventive role for curcumin in arterial diseases. In concordant with these findings are results of another study in which curcumin (10 mg) administered twice a day for 28 days lowered serum LDL and increased serum HDL levels in patients with atherosclerosis.[21] This effect could be explained on the basis of an enhanced excretion of cholesterol in bile by curcumin with a concomitant reduction in bile cholesterol saturation and elevated fecal fat excretion. New lines of investigation are being studied as to whether the hypocholesterolemic effect of turmeric is the result of a direct effect on liver or an indirect effect through thyroid hormones, since thyroid hormones affect reactions in almost all the pathways of lipid metabolism. Furthermore, it has been suggested that turmeric extract produces a decrease in triglyceride levels in human. Quercetin and quercetin monoglucoside (onion) inhibit 15-lipoxygenase dependent oxidation of LDL. Garlic and aged garlic extract (AGE) supplementation in humans has shown to protect oxidation of LDL. Ginger extract has shown to reduce plasma cholesterol levels and also significant reduction in the LDL basal oxidative state and susceptibility to oxidation in apolipoprotein E-deficient mice.

Garlic preparations have been shown to have antioxidant effects in vitro, in non-diabetic animals, and in humans. AGE and S-allylcysteine inhibits nitric oxide-induced intracellular oxidative stress in endothelial cells, inhibited LDL oxidation, and inhibited endothelial cell damage by oxidized LDL by directly scavenging intracellular peroxide and elevating the intracellular GSH content.[22,23] In humans, it was shown that the intake of garlic preparations for 2 weeks significantly decreased the oxidation of apolipoprotein B by 34%.[23] Administration of garlic oil and its sulfur-containing compounds increased the GSH content in red blood cells and the hepatic superoxide dismutase activity in nondiabetic rats.[24] Garlic oil was shown to reduce oxidative stress in diabetic rat model.[25] It was shown that LDL of healthy and type 2 diabetic subjects was protected from oxidation by several sulfur-containing compounds of garlic.[26,27] An anti-inflammatory effect of garlic was proposed in accordance with data from studies of garlic's anti-atherosclerotic and anti-tumorigenetic effects. Studies showed that the beneficial effects of garlic and its constituents may be due in part to its inhibitory effect on lipoxygenase, cyclooxygenase, and phospholipase A2, the enzymes involved in the generation of inflammatory prostaglandins and thromboxanes.[28,29] Recent studies suggested that garlic may suppress the expression of pro-inflammatory cytokines and iNOS upon activation of different immune cells.[30-32] In addition, it has also been reported that several garlic preparations can suppress the NFkB activation pathway. Regular consumption of chilli for 4 weeks increases the resistance of serum lipoproteins to oxidation.[33] Coriandrum sativum (Coriander) has been documented as a traditional treatment for cholesterol and diabetes patients. The seeds had a significant hypolipidemic action in rat model.[34] Thus, based on limited, but promising data, it appears that spices may exert beneficial effects in subjects with type 2 diabetes and CVD, and boost antioxidant defense mechanisms in healthy volunteers.

Platelet function

Platelet aggregation is accompanied by synthesis and release of pro-aggregatory molecules such as thromboxane (Tx) A_2 and ADP, which amplify platelet responses to collagen and recruit additional platelets to the site of injury.[4,35,36] The concerted action of collagen, ADP, and TxA_2 activates specific signaling pathways, generating a number of second messengers and leading to the functional expression of GPIIb-GPIIIa complex, the fibrinogen receptor on platelets.[4,35,36] Whereas pro-haemostatic mechanisms are counterbalanced and regulated by a number of physiologic anti-haemostatic molecules that work in a concerted and redundant manner, including the release of prostacyclin (PGI_2), nitric oxide, and endothelium-dependent hyperpolarizing factor by the endothelium as well as ADP hydrolyzing activity of endothelial cell membrane apyrase (CD39).[37-40] The aggregation of platelets by agonists is mediated, in part, through the intracellular formation of prostaglandin(PG) G_2, PGH_2 and TxA_2 from arachidonic acid,20:4n-6 (AA).[4,5,41,42] Non-nutritive compounds may have an important role in moderating AA metabolism and maintaining a healthy physiological state. In combination with n-3 fatty acids (fish oils) taken either as a dietary supplement or as a component of a balanced diet, they may offer a unique way to reduce AA-derived eicosanoid formation and to decrease the incidence of the chronic disorders such as CVD. In support of the pathophysiological role of platelets, platelet inhibitory drugs such as aspirin reduce the incidence of myocardial infarction, stroke and death from cardiovascular disease in secondary prevention trials.[43-45] Given the high incidence of cardiovascular disease in developed countries, there is still a great need for effective anti-platelet regimen. This concept has stimulated research into the prevention of platelet hyperactivity by several means including dietary supplementation. Dietary supplementation with AGE significantly inhibited both the total percentage and initial rate of platelet aggregation at concentrations of ADP up to 10 μmol/L.[46] No significant changes in plasma TxB_2 and 6-ketoPGF_{1a} concentrations or serum lipid profiles were observed. AGE, when taken as a dietary supplement by normolipidemic subjects, may be beneficial in protecting against CVD as a result of inhibiting platelet aggregation and lowering of plasma cholesterol. *Allium* spp. have provided a rich source of compounds which affect arachidonic acid (AA) metabolism. Conversely, methylallyltrisulphide from garlic oil, a potent inhibitor of platelet aggregation, promoted release of labelled AA from rabbit platelets implying stimulation of PLA_2. In this case labeled AA accumulated and the radiolabel was not found in prostanoids indicating inhibition at a later stage in the platelet AA cascade. Quercetin, a flavonol commonly encountered in food plants and a potent inhibitor of platelet aggregation is the only agent of dietary origin thought to directly inhibit phospholipase C.[47] Organosulphur compounds from *Allium* species, particularly *A. cepa* (onion) and *A. sativum* (garlic), have been shown to be potent inhibitors of platelet aggregation and to have antiasthmatic and antiallergic effects.[48,49] Most of the sulphur-containing compounds detected are formed from highly reactive sulphenic acids released from naturally-occurring S-alk(en)yl-L-cysteinesulphoxides by the action of alliin lyase (EC 4.4.1.4.-alliin alkyl-sulphenate-lyase) when tissues are damaged or disrupted.[50] Two groups of compounds predominate, the thiosulphinates, lachrymatory factors with demonstrable antiasthmatic activity *in vivo*[51] and the sulphinyldisulphides ("cepaenes") formed from the thiosulphinates by a mechanism similar to that described for the formation of the structurally-related (*E,Z*)-ajoene from allicin in garlic extracts.[52] Both groups of compounds have been shown to inhibit prostaglandin-endoperoxide synthase to varying extents.[51,53] Studies of the structure-activity relationships of the alpha-sulphinyldisulphides confirmed the requirement for sulphinyl and disulphide groups and showed that strength of inhibition of platelet aggregation was directly related to alkyl chain length with the propyl derivative showing greatest activity.[53] The activity of these structural variants against prostaglandin-endoperoxide synthase activity has not been reported but would be expected to parallel their capacity to inhibit platelet aggregation. Many extracts of food spices influence production of TXA_2 directly by inhibition of thromboxane A synthase and indirectly by inhibition of enzymes responsible for precursor formation.[54] A range of other compounds from spices and from the labiate herbs have been shown to inhibit prostaglandin endoperoxide synthase and otherwise influence prostanoid biosynthesis. A number of chalcones, including licochalcone A referred to above,[55] and the sweet-tasting triterpenoid from licorice, glycyrrhizin or its degradation product glycyrrhetic acid[56] have been reported to be mildly inhibitory of prostaglandin-endoperoxide synthase activity. Ginger (*Zingiber officinale*) extracts are also reported to be powerful inhibitors of human platelet aggregation and to inhibit prostanoid formation.[57,58] However the two effects do not appear directly related as [6]-gingerol and its analogues[59] reduce prostaglandin formation but are only weak inhibitors of platelet aggregation, whilst the labdane-type diterpenes from ginger strongly inhibit aggregation without inhibition of the arachidonic acid cascade. Evidently inhibition of aggregation requires a different mechanism from that of the organosulphur compounds derived from *Allium* sp..and it is suggested that the diterpenes mask the ADP binding site on platelets, inhibiting their activation.[60] The mechanism of inhibition of prostaglandin-endoperoxide synthase can be deduced from the relative effects of gingerol derivatives. Only methylgingerol, in which the phenolic hydroxyl is methylated, proved non-inhibitory confirming that the presence of a phenol group is essential. It is suggested that the phenol group inhibits radical formation or quenches radical generation in the prostaglandin-endoperoxide synthase reaction.[61] The hydrophobic alkyl side chains also play an important role by binding to the enzyme by hydrophobic interaction. Zingerone, a phenolic degradation product of gingerols in which the alkyl group is lost, was only weakly inhibitory compared to the parent gingerols. Gingerols with 6 or more alkyl carbons, in addition to inhibiting prostaglandin-endoperoxide synthase activity, were potent inhibitors of lipoxygenase. [6]-Gingerol, the main constituent responsible for the pungent taste of ginger, had an IC_{50} of 3.0 μM while the corresponding value for [10]-gingerol was approximately 0.05 μM. Further increase in alkyl chain-length up to 16 carbons did not improve potency.[62] Examination of structural variants of the phenolic function of the diarylheptanoids confirmed the earlier observation [58] that catechol (or guaiacyl) groups are essential to inhibitory action which operated through a radical scavenging or suppressing mechanism. Although the structure-function investigations made use of diarylheptanoids from a non-food source, related compounds are found in ginger,[60] turmeric and elsewhere. The link between inhibition of the arachidonic acid cascade with curcumin (and demethoxycurcumin and bis demethoxycurcumin) from turmeric (*Curcuma* spp.) and T-lymphocyte function has been demonstrated.

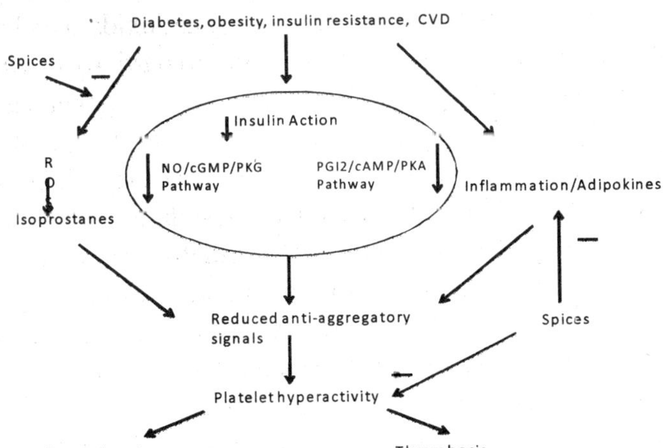

Figure 1. Mechanisms involved in the platelet hyperactivity in diabetes, obesity and insulin resistance

Aqueous extracts of coriander leaf, curry leaf, saffron, and cardamon inhibited platelet aggregation.[63] Aqueous extracts of several herbs also inhibited human platelet aggregation in vitro,[64] but human trials are not performed using these herbs. Tomato extract also inhibited both ADP and collagen induced aggregation up to 70% but could not inhibit arachidonic acid-induced platelet aggregation and concomitant thromboxane synthesis under similar experimental conditions.[65,13] Tomato contains very potent anti-platelet components, and consuming tomatoes might be beneficial both as a preventive and therapeutic regime for cardiovascular disease.

Conclusions

There is limited scientific evidence for the effects of spices on CVD and type 2 diabetes mellitus. More research is required, particularly examining the effects of chronic consumption patterns of the spices. With increasing interest in alternatives to non-steroidal anti-inflammatory agents in the management of chronic inflammation, and cardiovascular disease, research is emerging on the use of spices and herbs. Future consideration should be given to including more explicit recommendations about their place in a healthy diet. In addition to delivering antioxidant and other properties, spices can be used in recipes to partially or wholly replace less desirable ingredients such as salt, sugar and added saturated fat in, for example, marinades and dressings, stir-fry dishes, casseroles, soups, curries and Mediterranean-style cooking. As several metabolic diseases and age-related degenerative disorders are closely associated with oxidative processes in the body, the use of spices as a source of antioxidants to combat oxidation warrants further attention. Clinical trials with the spices should be carried out to establish their roles in the prevention of chronic diseases. From a dietary perspective, the functionality of spices will be exposed through consideration of their properties as foods. As with most foods, the real benefits of including them in the diet are likely to emerge with a better understanding of the attributes of health that are best supported by food, and in methodological developments addressing the evidence base for their effects. At present, recommendations are warranted to support the consumption of foods rich in bioactive components, such as herbs and spices. A greater body of scientific evidence is needed in supporting the benefits of spices in the overall maintenance of health and protection from disease.

References

1. H.C. Stary, *AJCN* **72,** 1297S–1306S (2000).
2. G.H. Gibbons, *Am J Cardiol* **79**, 3–8 (1997).
3. S. Toshima, A. Hasegawa, M: Kurabayashi. *Arterioscler. Thromb. Vasc. Biol.* **20**. 2243–2247 (2000).
4. A.K. Duttaroy, *Prost Leuk Essntl Fatty Acids*, **51**, 385-399(1994).
5. A.K. Duttaroy, T.K. Ray, A.K. Sinha, *Science,* **231**, 385-389 (1986).
6. M. Gawaz, *Cardiovasc Res*. **61**, 498- 511 (2004).
7. S. Massberg, Gawaz, M., Gruner, S., Schulte, V., Konrad, I., Zohlnhofer, D. U. Heinzmann, Nieswandt, B. *J Exp Med.* **197**, 41-49 (2003).
8. Z.M. Ruggeri, *Nat Med* **8** 1227-1234 (2002).
9. B.J. Willcox BJCurb JD, Rodriguez BL. *Am J Cardiol.* **101**, 75D-86D (2008).
10. L.A. Bazzano, J. He , L.G. Ogden, *Am. J. Clin .Nutr*. **76,** 93–99, (2002)
11. S. Liu, J.E. Manson, I-M. Lee I-M. *Am. J. Clin. Nutr*. **72**, 922–928.(2000).
12. A.K. Duttaroy, *Platelets*. **13**, 67-75 (2002).
13. N. O'Kennedy L. Crosbie, M. van Lieshout, J.I. Broom, D.J. Webb, A.K. Duttaroy *Am. J. Clin. Nutr*. **84**, 570-9 (2006).
14. L.C. Tapsell LC, Hemphill I, Cobiac L, Patch CS, Sullivan DR, Fenech M, Roodenrys S, Keogh JB, Clifton PM, Williams PG, Fazio VA, Inge KE. (2006) *Med. J. Aust* 185(4 Suppl), S4-24.
15. H.L. Madsen, B.R. Nielsen, G. Bertelsen, L.H. Skibsted , *Food Chem*. **57** 331–337(1996).

16. S. Shobana and K.A. Naidu, *Prostaglandins Leukot. Essent. Fatty acids* **62**, 107–110 (2000).

17. A.P. Reddy and Lokesh, B.R *Ann. Nutr. Metab.* 38, 343–358. (1994).

18. P. M. Kris-Etherton, K. D. Hecker, A. Bonanome, S. M. Coval, A.E. Binkoski, K. F. Hilpert, A.E. Griel, T. D Etherton , *Am J Med.* **113**, 71S– 88S (2002).

19. K. P. Kochar, *Indian J Physiol Pharmacol.* **52**, 106-122 (2008).

20. K. B. Soni , R. Kuttan, *Indian J Physiol Pharmacol* **36**, 273–275 (1992).

21. A. Ramirez Bosca, A. Soler, M. A. Carrion-Gutierrez, D. Pamies Mira, J. Pardo –Zapata, *J. Diaz-Alperi, Mech Ageing Dev* **114**, 207–210 (2000).

22. N. Ide, B. H. Lau, *J. Pharm. Pharmacol.* **49**, 908 – 911 (1997).

23. S. Phelps, W.S. Harris, *Lipids* **28**, 475 – 477 (1993).

24. L. Y. Sheen, H. W. Chen, Y.L. Kung, C.T. Liu, C.K., Lii, C. K., *Nutr. Cancer* , **35**, 160 –166 (1999).

25. M.M. Anwar, A.R. M.A Meki,*Comp. Biochem.* Physiol. A **135**, 539 – 547 (2003).

26. C.C. Ou, S.M. Tsao, M.C. Lin, M.C. Yin, *Lipids* **38,** 219 – 224 (2003).

27. C.N. Huang, J.S. Horng, M.C. Yin, *Agric. Food Chem.* **52**, 3674 – 3678 (2004).

28. M. Ali, M. Thomson, M. Afzal, *Prostaglandins Leukot. Essent. Fatty Acids* **62**, 55 – 73 (2000).

29. V.M. Dirsch, A.M. Vollmar, *Biochem. Pharmacol*, **61**, 587 – 593 (2001).

30. K.M. Kim, S.B. Chun, M.S. Koo, W.J. Choi, *Free Radic. Biol. Med.* **30**, 747 – 756 (2001).

31. G. Hodge, S. Hodge, P. Han, *Cytometry* **48**, 209 – 215 (2002).

32. H.P. Keiss, V.M. Dirsch, T. Hartung, T. Haffner, *J. Nutr.* **133**, 2171 – 2175(2003).

33. K. D. Ahuja KD, Ball MJ. *Br. J. Nutr.* **96**, 239-42(2006).

34. P. Dhanapakiam, J.M. Joseph, V.K. Ramaswamy, M., Moorthi A.S. Kumar. *J Environ. Biol.* **29**, 53-56.(2008).

35. M. H. Kroll, A.I. Schafer, *Blood,* **74**, 1181-1195 (1989).

36. B.S. Coller, K. Anderson, H.F. Weisman. *Thromb Haemost*, **74**: 302-308 (1995).

37. L.A. Harker, V. Fuster. *J. Am .Coll. Cardiol.* **8**: B21-B32 (1986).

38. A.K. Duttaroy, A.K. Sinha, *J Biol Chem.* **262**: 12685-12691 (1987).

39. B. Fisslthaler, R. Popp, L. Kiss, M. Potente, D.R. Harder, I. Fleming, R. Busse *Nature* **401**, 493-497 (1999).

40. A.K. Duttaroy, N.N. Kahn, A.K. Sinha. *Life Sci.* **49**, 1129-1139 (1991).

41. P. Hamet, S. Hidektasu, F. Umeda, D.J. Franks, *Metabolism* **32**, 124-130 (1983).

42. M.H. Kroll, A.I. Schafer, *Blood,* **74**: 1181-95 (1989).

43. S. Yusuf, J. Witties , I.J. Friedman I. *J. Am Med Assn.* **260**, 2259-63 (1988).

44. K. Schror . *Drugs* **50**, 7-28 (1995).

45. K. Schror, *Sem Thromb Haemost.* **23**: 349-356 (1997).

46. K. Rahman , D. Billington *J Nutr.* **130,** 2662-2665 (2000).

47. P. Pignatelli, F.M. Pulcinelli, A. Celestini , L. Lenti, A. Ghiselli, P.P. Gazzaniga, F.Violi . *Am. J.Clin. Nutr.* **72**, 1150-1115(2000).

48. K. C. Srivastava, *Prost. Leuk. Essntl. Fatty Acids*, **22**, 313-321 (1986).

49. K.C. Srivastava, O.D. Tyagi. *Prost Leuk Essntl Fatty Acids*, **49**, 587-595 (1993).

50. E. Block, S. Naganathan, D. Putman, S-H Zhao. *Pure & Appl Chem* **65**, 625-632 (1993).

51. T. Bayer, W. Brew, O. Seligman, V. Wray, H. Wagner. Phytochemist. **28**, 2373-2377 (1989).

52. E. Block, S. Ahmad, J.L. Catalfamo, M.K. Jain, R.J. Apitz-Castro. *Am. Chem. Soc.* **108**, 7045-7055 (1986).

53. S. Kawakishi, A. Morimitsu. Sulphur chemistry of onions and inhibitory factors of the arachidonic acid cascade. In: Food Phytochemicals for Cancer Prevention I (eds. Ho, C-T., Osawa, T., Huang, M-T., and Roscn, R.T.) pp. 120-127, ACS Symposium series 546, American Oil Chemical Society, Washington, DC, 1994.

54. J-H. Guh, F-N. Ko , T-T Jong, C-M Teng, *J Pharm Pharmacol* **47**, 329-332 (1995).

55. Y. Kimura, H. Okuda, T. Okuda , S. Arichi . *Phytotherpy Res* . **2**, 140-145 (1988).

56. Z.X. Wang, M. Nishioka, Y. Kurosaki, T. Nakayama, T. Kimura. *Biol Pharm Bull.* **18**, 1238-1241 (1995).

57. D.L. Flynn, M.F. Rafferty, A.M. Boctor. *Prost Leuk Med.* **24**, 195-198 (1986).

58. H. Kikuzaki, Y. Kawasaki, N. Nakatami. Structure of antioxidative compounds in ginger. In: Food Phytochemicals for Cancer Prevention I (eds. Ho, C-T., Osawa, T., Huang, M-T., and Rosen, R.T.) pp. 237-43, 1994, ACS Symposium series 546, American Oil Chemical Society, Washington, DC.

59. S. Kawakishi, A. Morimitsu, K. Koshimizu. Chemistry of ginger components and inhibitory factors of the arachidonic acid cascade. In: Food Phytochemicals for Cancer Prevention (eds. Ho, C-T., Osawa, T., Huang, M-T., and Rosen, R.T.) pp. 244-250, ACS Symposium series 546, American Oil Chemical Society, Washington, DC. 1994.

60. F. Kiuchi, S. Iwakami, M. Shibuya, F. Hanakoka, U. Sankawa. *Chem. Pharm . Bull* **40**, 387-391 (1992).

61. V. Misr, R.N. Misra, W.G. Unger, *Indian J Med Res.* **67**, 482-484 (1978).

62. K.C. Srivastava, A. Bordia, S.K. Verma, *Prost Leuk Essntl Fatty Acids* **52**, 223-227 (1995).

63. S.W. Jessie, T.P. Krishnakantha, *Pharmaceutical Biol.* **43**. 230-233 (2005).

64. S. Pierre, L. Crosbie , A.K. Duttaroy, *Platelets* **16**, 469-473 (2005).

65. A.K. Duttaroy, L.C. Crosbie, M.J. Gordon, *Platelets* **12,** 218-227 (2001).

Capsicum: A Medicinally Important Spice

Syed Ibrahim Rizvi and Suaib Luqman

Capsicum refers to the fruits of several species belonging to Solanaceae family. Capsicum is especially popular in hot climates where its normal dietary intake may be as high as 2.5 grams per day. It has been intriguing for scientists to explain why consumption of capsicum is high in hot climatic regions of the world. Folk uses of capsicum include apetite stimulation, treatment of gastric ulcers and rheumatism, and restoration of hair growth. It is also known to help in 'cold' rheumatic and arthritic conditions, diphtheria, tonsillitis and diarrhea. The pungent principle in chillies is an alkaloid (vanilloid) called capsaicin. The neuronal effect of capsaicin has been intensively investigated. Capsaicin also displays many non-neuronal effects which are either due to non-specific action of this lipophilic molecule on the plasma membrane or due to antioxidant effect. Despite a huge amount of research, the physiological implication of increased consumption of capsicum in hot climatic regions remains unclear.

Introduction

Capsicum refers to the fruits of several species belonging to Solanaceae family. The term CAPSICUM is derived either from the Greek word "Kapso" meaning to bite or from the Latin "Capsa" meaning box. Capsicum is especially popular in hot climates where its normal dietary intake may be as high as 2.5 grams per day.[1] It has been intriguing for scientists to explain why consumption of capsicum is high in hot climatic regions of the world. Oral consumption of capsicum causes profuse perspiration, termed gustatory sweating.[2] This effect leads to heat loss which is clearly beneficial "side effect" in hot climates.

The worldwide popularity of chillies has prompted numerous investigations of the biologic properties of capsaicin, yet its evolutionary significance in the plants that produce them remained unclear for long. Chillies are low shrubs with fruit that is accessible to mammals as well as birds. However, capsaicin in the fruit has been found to repel or poison mammals but not birds.[3] This taxonomic distinction is predicted by the 'direct deterrence' (toxicity) hypothesis, whereby capsaicin in ripe fruits selectively discourages vertebrate predators without deterring birds which are more effective seed dispersers.[4]

Hot peppers have been used as a condiment as well as for food. They are used as flavoring agents, and coloring material in cookery. It is employed as an additive to native foods. Tabasco sauce is made by pickling the pulp in strong vinegar and / or brine. Oil of pepper is valued as a flavouring for sausages, canned meats, soups, table sauces, certain beverages and liquors. *Capsicum frutescens* is used in the manufacture of sauces and curry powders and also in preparations of pickles. *Capsicum annuum*, the green non-pungent form are eaten raw as salads. The colouring matter of the ripe fruit consists of several compounds such as - Capsanthin, capsorubin, zeaxanthin, lutein, cryptoxanthin, α and β carotenes and a few unidentified xanthophylls.

History and Traditional uses of capsicum

Capsicum has been known since the beginning of civilization in the Western Hemisphere. It has been a part of the human diet since about 7500 BC.[5] Chilli is historically associated with the voyage of Columbus.[6] Columbus is given credit for introducing chilli to Europe, and subsequently to Africa and to Asia. On his first voyage, he encountered a plant whose fruit mimicked the pungency of the black pepper, *Piper nigrum* L. Columbus called it red pepper because the pods were red. Capsicum is not related to the Piper genus. In 1493, Peter Martyr[7] wrote that Columbus brought home "pepper more pungent than that from the Caucasus." Chilli spread rapidly across Europe into India, China, and Japan. The new spice was incorporated into the cuisines instantaneously. Probably for the first time, pepper was no longer a luxury spice only the rich could afford. Since its discovery by Columbus, chilli has been incorporated into most of the world's cuisines.

The medicinal use of Capsicum antedates the discovery of New World: it was used by Native Americans to cure cramps as well as diarrhea. Other folk uses of Capsicum include apetite stimulation, treatment of gastric ulcers and rheumatism, and restoration of hair growth.[8] Capsicum is known for stimulating the circulation and altering temperature regulation and is also used in high fevers. Applied to the skin, Capsicum paste, desensitizes nerve endings and it has been used in the past as a local analgesic. The capsicidins found in the seeds of capsicum fruits are believed to have antibiotic properties. The heating quality of capsicum makes it a valuable remedy for poor circulation and related conditions. In particular, it improves blood flow to the hands and feet and to the central organs.[9]

The uses of capsicum in traditional medicines are multifold.[10] It is also rubefacient, increasing blood flow to the affected parts and this helps to stimulate the circulation in 'cold' rheumatic and arthritic conditions, aiding the removal of waste products and increasing the flow of nutrients to the tissues. A paste of capsicum is used locally in tonsilities. In diphtheria its application believed to hasten cure. Chillies are taken to relieve wind and colic and to stimulate secretion of the digestive juices, thereby aiding digestion. A pinch of chilly powder is excellent in gargles for sore throats. Finally, extraordinary as it may seem, chillies are useful for some types of diarrhea. Capsicum in combination with cinchona is used in gout and advanced stages of rheumatism. Capsicum has also been used as a remedy for snake-bite.[11]

Role of Capsicum in amelioration of learning impairment has been documented. The effect of dietary red bell pepper (*Capsicum annum* L.) on learning performance was studied in the senescence-accelerated mouse (SAM). It was observed that SAMP8 mice that received diet supplemented with red bell pepper powder showed much better acquisition in passive avoidance tasks as compared with the control groups.[12]

The role of capsicum consumption has been reported to influence carbohydrate metabolism in humans.[13] Aqueous extracts of *Capsicum* sp. have been reported to display significant antimicrobial effects.[14]

Capsaicin: A Hot Tool

The pungent principle in chillies is an alkaloid (vanilloid) called capsaicin. Capsaicin is a crystalline condensation product of 3-hydroxy-4-methoxy benzylamine and decylenic acid, which produces a highly irritating vapour on heating. Capsaicin retains its pungency in a dilution of one in a million parts of water. Its content varies from 0.0 - 1.8 percent in different capsicum species. Commercial chilli samples contain about 0.1 per cent capsaicin.

The chemical properties of capsaicin have been extensively investigated.[15] It is weakly acidic, and contains a phenolic group as shown in Figure 1.

Figure 1

Structure of capsaicin (*trans* – 8-methyl-*N*-vanillyl – 6-nonenamide)

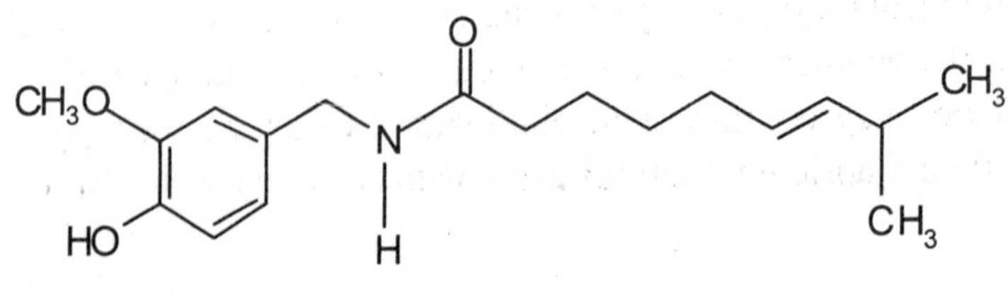

Formula	:	$C_{18}H_{27}O_3N$
Formula weight	:	305.4
Nomenclature	:	trans 8-methyl-N-vanillyl-6-nonenamide
Melting point	:	64° - 65°C
Boiling point	:	210° - 220°C
Solubility	:	Capsaicin is sparingly soluble in cold water and more soluble in boiling water but readily soluble in organic solvent like ethanol, acetone and chloroform.

It is not precipitated, or only very slightly, by the usual reagents which precipitate alkaloids. The phenolic group can be methylated to form methyl capsaicin, a derivative with much less pungency than the parent compound.

The pungency of capsaicin is measured in Scoville Heat Units (SHU). In 1912, Wilbur Scoville calibrated the potency of pepper by extracting capsicum in alcohol and diluting it until pungency was just detected after placing a drop on his tongue. The threshold concentrations of capsaicin that produce a lukewarm and painful, burning sensation on the tongue arc 2 x 10^7 and > 10^{-6} g/ml respectively.[16] Nowadays, the pungency of chillies with their capsaicin content are analysed by using HPLC . Other methods used to measure pungency include colorimetry, which however, gives errors due to interference by other colouring principles. Thin layer chromatography has also been used. A chain of biochemical and physiological reactions that generates a heat sensation accompanies the pungency of capsaicin. We now know that this capsaicin-produced heat sensation may have broader effect on our bodies than just a pleasant sensory perception. The 'hot' taste of capsaicin may add nutritive value to the foods by enhancing the bioavailability of vital nutrients.

SHU of some of the chillies with their content- capsaicin, dihydrocapsaicin are given in **Table 1**.

Table - 1

Capsaicin and Dihydrocapsaicin content and pungency in different varieties of Indian red chillies[17]

Capsicum Type	Capsaicin (% w/w)	Dihydrocapsaicin (% w/w)	Pungency (SHU)
Tezpur	4.28	1.42	855000
Guntur	0.20	0.16	53250
Gwalior	0.43	0.23	112500
Kashmir	0.18	0.09	40500
Patna	0.44	0.21	96000

India's BHUT JOLOKIA has been confirmed as the hottest chilli variety by The Guiness Book of Records with 1001304 Scoville Heat Units. It is a naturally occuring hybrid native to the Assam region of north eastern India. Prior to this, Tezpur chilli variety (855000 SHU) and Red Savina Habanero, a mexican variety (577000 SHU) was reported to be the hottest chilli in the world.[17]

Neuronal effects of capsaicin

Capsaicin binds to a sub class of sensory neurons that carry sensation of pain. These neurons, called nociceptors, transmit information regarding tissue damage to pain processing centres in the spinal cord and brain. In mammals, exposure of nociceptor terminals to capsaicin leads initially to excitation of the neuron and the consequent perception of pain and local release of inflammatory mediators. With prolonged exposure, nociceptor terminals become insensitive to capsaicin, as well as to other noxious stimuli.[18] Nociceptor desensitisation has been exploited for the use of capsaicin as an analgesic agent in the treatment of painful disorders ranging from viral and diabetic neuropathies to rheumatoid arthritis.[19]

Electrophysiological and biochemical studies have shown that capsaicin excites nociceptors by increasing the permeability of the plasma membrane to cations.[20] Later studies proved that upon binding to nociceptors, capsaicin activates an ion channel that allows calcium ions to flow from outside the cell (where its concentration is 2 mM) into the intracellular space (where the concentration of calcium is very low: 100 nM).[21]

Non-neuronal effects of capsaicin

The acute actions of capsaicin, however, are not restricted to neurons, and there are a number of reports of capsaicin influencing non-neural systems. These cell non-selective effects of capsaicin and capsaicin congeners include: inhibition of cardiac muscle excitability,[22] inhibition of visceral smooth muscle activity[23] and contraction of vascular smooth muscle.[24] An interesting observation is that capsaicin can inhibit the growth of a number of transformed cell lines.[25] Capsaicin also inhibits the plasma membrane electron transport system and induces apoptosis in transformed cells.[26] The finding suggests that the plasma membrane electron transport system may be an interesting target to design anti-tumor and anti-inflammatory drugs.

Due to its lipophilic nature capsaicin can partition within lipid bilayers. This activity has the potential to alter membrane fluidity, redox state, and lipid-protein interaction. Capsaicin has been reported to alter plasma membrane structure and fluidity in a concentration dependent manner.[27] The role of capsaicin in modulating the activity of human erythrocyte membrane bound Na/K-ATPase and Ca^{2+}-ATPase[28] and acetylcholinesterase activity[29] has also been reported. The physiological implications of these alterations are however[30] not yet understood.

Several studies report the presence of antioxidant activity in capsaicin.[31-34] The compound has been shown to protect erythrocytes from oxidative stress, treatment with capsaicin has been shown to reduce protein oxidation and lipid peroxidation [35] in oxidatively stressed human erythrocytes. Importantly capsaicin and its analogues were found to be devoid of pro-oxidant activity and showed a highly significant antioxidant activity in all systems investigated. The antioxidant activity present in capsaicin suggests that in addition to imparting flavor to the food, capsicum has potential health benefits associated with antioxidant defense.

Current uses of Capsaicin and future perspectives

In principle, all the three characteristic actions of capsaicin (excitation, desensitization and neurotoxicity) may have therapeutic value.[36] Stimulation (counter - irritation) and desensitization are already in use in clinical practice. Capsaicin is classified by the FDA as a counter irritant, a substance which may be deliberately applied to the skin to relieve irritation and pain. It is a standard ingredient in a variety of over the counter drugs used world wide to relieve muscle ache. This effect of capsaicin serves as the basis for its use as a valuable tool in investigating the roles of sensory neurons in biological functions.[37]

Conclusion

It remains a mystery why is it that the same hot taste of capsicum which repels a variety of mammals from rats to squirrel to dogs, is found pleasurable by humans. Psychologists speculate that eating hot peppers might be a form of masochism. This theory is however at variance with the well-known geographic pattern of hot peppers consumption, namely, people living in tropical climates prefer their food hotter than those residing in temperate climates. This may be due to the fact that eating hot and spicy food helps combat the warm climate via gustatory sweating. Nonetheless, the human liking or aversion towards the taste of hot peppers is probably far more complex than this simple physiological implication.

References

1. J. A. Rumsfield and D. P. West, *DICP Ann. Pharmacother.* **25,** 381 (1991).

2. T. S. Lee, *J. Physiol.* **124,** 528 (1954).

3. J. R. Mason, N. J. Bean, P. S. Shah and I. Clark, *J. Chem. Biol.* **17,** 2539 (1991).

4. J. J. Tewksbury and G. P. Nabhan, *Nature* **412,** 403 (2001).

5. R. S. MacNeish, *Science* **143,** 531 (1964).

6. C. B. Heiser, The evolution of crops plants (ed. Simmonds), p. 265 (1976) (Longman Press, London).

7. J. Andrews, Peppers: the domesticated *Capsicum*s, (1984) (Univ. of Texas Press, Austin, TX).

8. T. D. Whittet, *Proc. Royal Soc. Med.* **61,** 801 (1968).

9. A. Szallasi, *Acta Physiol. Scand.* **155,** 1 (1995).

10. A. K. Nadkarni, Indian Materia Medica, Vol. 1. pp 269 (1976) (Popular Prakashan Pvt. Ltd. Bombay, India).

11. F. Lembeck, *Acta Physiol. Hung.* **69,** 265 (1987).

12. H. Suganuma, T. Hirano and T. Inakuma, *J. Nutr. Sci. Vitaminol.* **45 (1),** 143 (1999).

13. K. Lim, M. Yoshioka, S. Kikuzato, A. Kiyonaga, H. Tanaka, M. Shindo and M. Suzuki, *Med. Sci. Sports Exerc.* **29 (3),** 355 (1997).

14. R. H. Cichewicz and P.A. Thorpe, *J. Ethnopharmacol.* **52 (2),** 61 (1996).

15. V. S. Govindrajan, *CRC Crit.Rev.Food Sci. & Nutr.* **22 (2),** 108 (1985).

16. J. Szolcsanyi, Pyretics and Anti-pyretics Vol. 60, p. 347 (Springer-Verlag Berlin).

17. R. Mathur, R. S. Dangi, S. C. Dass and R. C. Malhotra, *Curr. Sci.* **79 (3),** 287 (2000).

18. J. Szolcsanyi, in Capsaicin in the study of Pain (ed. J. N. Wood), p. 1(1993) (Academic Press, San Diego, CA).

19. A. Szallasi and P. M. Blumberg, *Pharmacol. Rev.* **51 (2),** 159 (1999).

20. I. F. James, N. N. Ninkina, J. N. Wood, in Capsaicin in Study of Pain (ed. J. N. Wood), p. 83, (1993) (Academic, London).

21. A. Dray, C. A. Forbes and G. M. Burges, *Neurosci. Letter* **110,** 52 (1990).

22. A. Franco-Cereceda, J. M. Lundberg, A. Saria, W. Schreibmayer and H. A. Tritthart, *Acta Physiol. Scand.* **132,** 181 (1990).

23. M. Takaki, J. G. Jin, Y. F. Lu and S. Nakayama, *Eur. J. Pharmacol.* **186**, 71 (1990).

24. P. Holzer, *Pharmacol. Rev.* **43**, 143 (1991).

25. D. J. Moore, P. J. Chuheh and D. M. Moore, *Proc. Natl. Acad. Sci. USA* **92,** 1831 (1995).

26. A. Macho, M. A. Calzado, J. Munoz-Blanco, C. Gomez-Diaz, F. Mollinedo, P. Navas and E. Munoz, *Cell Death Differ*. **6,** 155 (1999).

27. H. Tsuchiya, *J.Ethnopharmacol.* **75**, 295 (2001).

28. S.I.Rizvi and S.Luqman, *Cell. Mol. Biol. Lett.* **8**,919, (2003).

29. A.K.De, D.Sengupta and J.J.Ghosh, *Phytother. Res.* 7, 310 (1993).

30. S.I.Rizvi and S.Luqman, *Med. Chem. Res.* **10**, 502 (2001).

31. M.Materska and I. Perucka, *J. Agric. Food Chem.* **53,** 1750 (2005).

32. A.Rosa, M.Delana, V.Casu, S.Paccagnini, G.Appendino, M.Ballero and M.A. Dessi, *J. Agric. Food. Chem.* **50**, 7396 (2002).

33. S. I. Rizvi and S. Luqman, *Med. Chem. Res.* **11**, 301 (2002).

34. S. Luqman and S. I. Rizvi, *Oxid. Commun.* **33**, 430 (2010).

35. S.Luqman and S.I.Rizvi, *Phytother. Res.* **20**, 303 (2006).

36. A. Szallasi and P.M.Blumberg, *Adv. Pharmacol.* **24**, 123 (1993).

37. S.H. Buck, M.S.Miller and T.F.Burks, *Brain Res.* **233,** 216 (1982).

Trends in Chilli Breeding

Indira,P., Pradeepkumar,T ; Sadhan kumar, P. G and Peter, K.V.

Chilli is a vegetable cum spice. Originated in South America it spread to allover the world. India possesses rich diversity in chillies. Chilli being treated as a field crop, productivity is low in addition to susceptibility to diseases like wilt, leaf curl, rots and leaf spots. Being often cross pollinated mass selection is used to upgrade productivity. Heterosis has been exploited and several F1 hybrids are now released. Interspecific hybridization has been resorted to incorporate desirable traits. Mutation breeding has been resorted to eliminate undesirable traits. Research by private seed companies has given good dividents. Several improved varieties and hybrids are now available.

Introduction

Chilli is a unique spice cum vegetable crop of commercial importance in India. Green chilli, Chilli pepper, cayenne pepper, Tabasco, paprika, sweet/bell pepper, pimentos, serrano pepper, are all derived from the fruit of different species of *Capsicum* .The pungent types are used as green chilli, whole dry chilli ,chilli powder, chilli paste, chilli sauce, chilli oleoresin and as mixed powder.

Though chilli is grown throughout India, Andhra Pradesh, Maharashtra, Karnataka and Tamil Nadu account for about 75per cent of total area and annual production in India. However among the chilli growing Indian states, Andhra Pradesh and Punjab ranks top in average yield . But the average yield in India (1ton\ha) is low as compared to USA, S.Korea and Japan(3-4tons\ha).[1] Main reasons for low yield are low coverage of high yielding varieties/ hybrids, heavy incidence of pests and diseases and lack of adoption of scientific package of practices in cultivation.

Though Chilli is not a commercial crop in Kerala, its cultivation is restricted to certain tracts. But many land races like white kanthari, Green chuna, Neymulagu etc. are popular among the farmers as green chilli. As they are shade tolerant they are suitable for intercropping in homestead gardens of Kerala, especially during rainy season. But dry chilli cultivation is not much feasible due to high rainfall and the consequent occurrence of many fungal diseases like fruit rot,leaf spot etc. during rainy season.

Chilli cultivation in the acidic soils of Kerala is limited due to the incidence of bacterial wilt and chilli mosaic /leaf curl complex during summer season also. These two diseases are the main threats for commercial cultivation of dry chilli in Kerala during summer.

Bacterial wilt Disease

Bacterial wilt caused *by Ralstonia solanacearum* (Smith) Yabuchi *et al* is one of the most destructive plant diseases in the warm humid region of the world. This is a major constraint for chilli cultivation in Kerala,Orissa,Goa,Andaman and Nicobar Islands and Coastal Districts of Tamil Nadu,Andhra Pradesh and West Bengal.

The state of Kerala is a warm humid tropical region having a mean maximum and minimum temperature of 33^{0}C and 24^{0}C respectively and relative humidity more than 80 per cent. Rainfall is around 300cm and mean soil temperature varies with soil depth ranges from 27^{0}C and 36^{0}C.Kerala has different soil types like red loam, laterite, sandy, alluvial, forest loam and black soils which are of acidic and alkaline nature. The above soil plant atmosphere continuum is favourable to the incidence of bacterial wilt in Kerala.[2]

Breeding for disease resistance is the major avenue for the control of bacterial wilt diseases. Successful control of bacterial wilt of solanaceous vegetables is achieved through development and use of resistant varieties in Kerala.

A total of 150 genotypes belonging to three species viz. *C. annuum, C. chinense and C.frutescens* was screened for resistance to bacterial wilt in an ICAR Adhoc scheme on "Breeding for resistance to bacterial wilt in chilli and brinjal"at Vellanikkara, Trichur. In general wilt incidence was minimum in *C. chinense a*ccessions and maximum in *C. annuum*. Two clustered *C. annuum* accessions CA 33 and CA 219 were resistant to bacterial wilt.[1] Fifty one chilli genotypes evaluated in another ICAR Adhoc scheme on "Heterosis breeding in chilli and brinjal associated with resistance to bacterial wilt" also confirmed the wilt resistance of CA 33 and CA 219. These clustered accessions were further improved through single plant selection. CA 33-1-4-6 was recommended by the KAU variety evaluation committee for wilt prone areas under the name Manjari. It has small fruits (4cm) of light green colour which are born in clusters.

CA 219 was released by the State seed sub committee on crop standards under the name **"Ujwala".** It has longer fruits (6-7 cm) which are dark green in colour in immature stage turing deep red on ripening. Fruits are valued for high pungency and colour value. It is an ideal variety for pot culture because of its compact growth and attractive fruits and is free from leaf curl and mosaic diseases.

Ten hybrids were evaluated along with pant C 1 and Manjari for bacterial wilt reaction along with susceptible check, Hungarian wax, Yolo Wonder Improved. Manjari was moderately resistant (33.30%).[2]

Near isogenic lines were developed lines by crossing Ujwala and Pusa Jwala.[3] The resistant plants of BC_2 generation resulted from cross of BC_1 and Pusa Jwala were selfed to produce BC_2F_2.

Bacterial wilt resistant plants having characteristics of Pusa Jwala were selected and used in the initial material for producing near isogenic lines of Pusa Jwala having resistance to bacterial wilt. They were further advanced to BC_2F_8 generation CA 752 a near isogenic line at BC_2F_8 was stabilized for yield and resistance to bacterial wilt and was released under the name **Anugraha**.

Studies on biochemical basis of resistance to bacterial wilt revealed that total phenol, OD phenol, proteins contents and enzyme activities had positive association with resistance. The wilt resistant variety Ujwala had higher OD phenol and protein contents on inoculation while susceptible variety had high total phenol content .Both peroxidase and polyphenol oxidase activity were higher in resistant variety than in susceptible one. The higher amount of OD phenol and their oxidation products like quinones formed by increased peroxidase and polyphenol oxidase were ascribed for resistance in Ujwala.

A single incompletely dominant gene inherited resistance to bacterial wilt in Ujwala. In radiotracer studies, radioactivity counts were more in susceptible variety than in resistant one after inoculation in both 32p and 35s labelled plants. In the auto radiography, the 35s labelled bacteria were more in susceptible plants than in resistant ones.

Chilli mosaic

Mosaic disease of *Capsicum* was wide spread in commercially cultivated fields in Karnataka with disease incidence ranging from 11.8-94.8 % with an average of 53%.The first report on mosaic diseases of pepper in India was from the erst while Bombay Province.[4-5] Later several viruses causing mosaic on bell pepper and chilli have been reported by many scientists.

Out of the eighteen viruses reported to occur naturally on pepper throughout the world, only ten have been reported from India viz. Tobacco leaf curl virus,[6] Indian chilli mosaic virus,[7] Potato virus X,[8] Cucumber mosaic virus,[9] Potato virus Y, Tobacco ring spot virus,[10] Pepper veinal mottle virus, Pepper vein banding virus and Tobacco etch virus.[11]

Morphological aspects of four F_1 hybrids of crosses involving Local Blue as seed parent and Russian, Indian Long Red, Chinese Giant and Oskosh as pollen parents were studied.[12] All the F_1 s, like the common seed parent Local Blue, exhibited resistance against mosaic diseases.

Based on symptomatology and indicator plant method, the isolates collected from different parts of Kerala were identified as potato virus Y (PVY). Serological method and electron microscopy confirmed the identify of the isolates. The chilli lines CA 10, CA 52, CA 48, CA 47 and Local Blue were found tolerant to leaf curl complex at College of Agriculture, Vellayani during 1985-86.

One hundred and fourteen genotypes belonging to different species were screened for resistance to mosaic virus in an ICAR Adhoc scheme on "Breeding for resistance to mosaic virus in chilli." Eleven genotypes were found resistant and 21 tolerant. The eleven genotypes viz. CA 109 (Tam mild Jalapeno) CA 107 (Hidalgo serrano), CA 108 (Tam mild chile -2) CA 118, (IHR-384),CA 119 (IHR 517-1),CA 121(koppam Local)Pusa Jwala , CA 138 (PI 163201) Pusa Sadabahar, CA-142(Tumpang) and CA-144(L. 2722) were found resistant to mosaic virus in the preliminary screening under different seasons.[13]

Out of the 53 accessions tested the accessions CA 337, CA 731,CA 738, CA 739, and CA 744 possessed resistance to both bacterial wilt and mosaic.[14] The F_1s developed using the resistant parents were found susceptible to both bacterial wilt and mosaic.Chilli varieties Punjab Lal, Lorai, PBC 142,and PBC 204 were also found resistant to mosaic diseases.

Field screening of the 37 cultivars for leaf curl resistance revealed tolerance in eight genotypes, susceptibility in 27 and high susceptibility in two.[15] Mangalapuram Local was identified as a desirable accession as it produced high yield in spite of the diseases.

In another screening trial against leaf curl diseases, plants infected were screened on 45th day after transplanting. The percentage of infected plants were 47.5% in Pusa Jwala, 17.5% in G_4,47% in K2, 100% in CA 89 and 20 % in cluster The PVY mosaic resistance was confirmed as monogenic recessive in nature.

Screening against root knot nematode

Ten varieties of chilli were screened against root knot nematode at AICVIP, Vellanikkara,Thrissur. Four were resistant (CA 70-A, CA 2057, CA 2210, CA 2104) four moderately resistant (CA2109, CA1068, CA 2123, and CA 2023) and two susceptible. Chuna,CA 33, Pant C_1, and White Kanthari were found resistant.

Abiotic stresses

There are many environmental factors like high and low temperature, drought, excessive moisture, salinity, atmospheric pollutants and minerals in the soil which affect crop production . Among these drought, temperature, salinity etc. are some of the stresses affecting chilli production.

Drought Tolerance

The ability of a plant to withstand low tissue water potential may be considered as drought tolerance. Drought tolerance was observed in *Capsicum cardenasii,*[16] and in *C. chacoense.* It was reported that the mean stomatal density *C. chacoense* is only 174.67 (per mm^2) when compared to *C. annuum* (185.58/mm^2). Deep root system of *C.chacoense* also favours drought tolerance.[17]

Shade tolerance

Though chilli is not a commercial crop of Kerala , many land races are grown in the homesteads as an intercrop in coconut garden to meet the daily requirement of green chilli .They are mostly grown in rainy season ,due to heavy incidence of pests during summer. Some of the land races are perennial and shade tolerant also.

The physiological, anatomical, biochemical and genetic basis of shade tolerance were analyzed.[18] Seventy genotypes belonging to *C.annuum, C. frutescens* and *C.chinense* were evaluated under 25,50 and 75 percent shade in comparison with open condition.CA 38 of *C.annuum* CF 51 of *C. frutescens* and CC63 of *C. chinense* were identified as shade tolerant and CA 39 of *C. annuum* ,CF 46 of *C.frutescens* and CC66 of *C. chinense* as shade susceptible genotype.

Genotypes grown under open condition had thicker leaves with more stomata per unit area. The upper and lower epidermal cells, palisade and spongy mesophyll cells and vascular bundle thickness were maximum in open. The increase in chlorophyll a, b and total chlorophyll under shade was prominent in shade tolerant genotypes. A decreasing trend was observed in chlorophyll a/b ratio in all the genotypes. The shade tolerant genotypes were found to maintain higher protein and total phenol content under shade. Capsaicin, oleoresin and ascorbic acid content did not vary significantly due to shade. Under open condition the genotype recorded higher cartenoid content. A polygenic system of inheritance with non allelic interaction was revealed in shade tolerance. Duplicate type of epistasis with additive additive x additive, dominance and dominance x dominance components of genetic variance were also observed. A high yielding, early maturing variety with low attractive medium pungent fruits having excellent acceptability as green chilli tolerant to partial shade was released as **Vellayani Athulya**.

Selection involving F_2 toF_5 generation of crosses Pant C_1 x Purple cluster, G_4 x Pusa Jwala and Vellanotchi x Pusa Jwala were conducted at the College of Agriculture, Vellayani .This resulted in the development of two less pungent chilli varieties, **Jwala Mukhi** and **Jwala Sakhi** through recombination breeding between Pusa Jwala and Vellanotchi .Jwala Mukhi can grow and yield well even under partial shade .Both of them are suitable for cultivation in the red soil of the South Kerala.

Quality evaluation

Colour value

Chilli fruits exhibited highest colour values at full ripe stage and lowest at turning stage. The fruits were least pungent when harvested at turning stage and the pungency showed an increasing trend as the harvesting was progressed from turning to full ripe and withering stage. Most of the green fruited accessions of *Capsicum frutescens* had higher carotenoid content as compared to white fruited types. Green and yellow coloured oleoresin was obtained from *C. frutescens* green and white types respectively. The accessions studied could be classified based on capsaicin content as high (1-1.5%), medium (0.25-0.75%) and low (0.11-0.25). The bird pepper accessions exhibited significant variations in ascorbic acid content at both stages of maturity. It ranged from 21.00-77.6 mg/100g in mature frits and 31.5-135.75 mg/100g and 71.6 mg/100g respectively.[19]

Oleoresin content

Nine genotypes belonging to different species were evaluated in three seasons *viz.,* summer, rainy and winter for oleoresin yield using ethyl acetate.[20] Maximum % of oleoresin was estimated in Arka Lohit (32.43), KTPL- 19 had the highest oleoresin % (37.83) during winter. The oleoresin extracted from the variety Ujwala was subjected to storage study in four types of containers. The type of container did not influence the colour loss. The oleoresin stored in dark was higher in colour value compared to samples kept in open. Storage is not advisable for colour retention. For capsaicin open condition was better than dark storage. Delaying the harvest to withering stage and storing the oleoresin in polythene containers for 8 months under open conditions can be recommended for increased pungency.[20]

References

1. T.R Gopalakrishnan ,.(ed). Three decades of vegetable Research in Kerala Agricultural University. Kerala Agricultural University (2004).
2. Girijaderi Intervarietal heterosis in *C.annuum* and evaluation of set of clustered bell peppers . M.Sc. (Hort) thesis, Kerala Agricultural University, Thrissur, Kerala, (1986).
3. B.L Markose,. Genetic and biochemical basis of resistance to bacterial wilt in chilli Ph.D (Hort) thesis, Kerala Agricultural University, Thrissur, Kerala, (1996).
4. W.Mcrae, Economic Botany part III mycology A. Rep. Bd Sci, Advice India **23**:31-35, (1924).
5. G.S Kulkarni,. *Poona agric. coll. Mag.* **16**:6-12. (1924).
6. R.S Vasudeva ,. *Scient. Rep. agric. Res.* .**53**:79-89. (1954).
7. A Jha, and S.P Raychaudhari, *Indian J. Agricultural Science* **26**:217-222. (1956).
8. Kandaswamy, T.K., Janaki, I.P., Ramakrishan, K., Thangamani,G., Raju, S.K.T. and Sellamani, S. *Madras agric J.* 50-110, (1963).
9. A.Anjaneyulu, and A Apparao, *Indian phytopath.* **20** :380-381, (1967).
10. E.Jeyarajan, and K Ramakrishan, *Madras agric. J.***56**:761-766. (1996).
11. V.B. Bidari, Distribution and epidemiology of chilli viruses in Karnataka Ph. D. thesis, University of Agricultural Sciences, Bangalore. (1982).
12. Nair Cytomorphological and chemical studies on inter varietal crosses of *C.annuum* L. M.C. Agricultural COA. (1970).
13. T.E George, Final Research report of ICAR Adhoc scheme on Breeding for resistance to mosaic viruses in chilli. *Capsicum annuum* L RARS, Pattambi. (1998).
14. A.G Fatima, Screening of chilli(*C.annuum* L.) genotypes for resistance to bacterial wilt and mosaic. M.Sc. (Hort) thesis, Kerala Agricultural University, Thrissur, Kerala. (1999).
15. L Jose, Genetic variability in chilli (*C.annuum* L.) with emphasis to reaction to leaf curl virus, M.Sc. thesis, Kerala Agricultural University, Thrissur, Kerala (2007).

16. B Pickersgill, Some aspects of interspecific hybridization in capsicum. Paper presented during fourth meeting of Eucarpia capsicum working group, 14-16 October,1980, Wageningen, Netherlands. (1980).

17. T Pradeepkumar, Interspecific hybridization in capsicum.M.Sc thesis. Rao, P.R.D.V.J.1976.Characterization and identification of some chilli mosaic viruses. Ph .D thesis, University of Agricultural Sciences, Bangalore. (1990).

18. I Sreelathakumari, *Horticulture* 7: 41-52. (2000).

19. K. B Sheela, Genetic improvement of bird pepper (*Capsicum frutescens* L.) by selection. Ph. D. Thesis, Kerala Agricultural University, Thrissur, Kerala. (1998).

20. C. Mini, Oleoresin recovery, quality characterization and storage stability in chilly (*Capsicum* Spp.) genotypes. Ph. D. Thesis, Kerala Agricultural University, Thrissur, Kerala. (1997).

Cardamom–Botany and Horticulture: A Review

V A Parthasarathy, V Srinivasan, D Prasath and K N Shiva

Cardamom (Elettaria cardamomum Maton), is an important spice crop and is native of evergreen forests of Western Ghats of South India. In spite of its prominence in world trade from time immemorial, cardamom received much attention in the second half of this century. This review highlights achievements in cardamom breeding and production technologies. The scope of the discussion addresses origin, chemistry, medicinal and pharmacology, botany, genetic resources, breeding methods, biotechnological approaches and horticulture aspects of crop production.

Introduction

Cardamom of commerce, popularly known as "Queen of Spices" is the dried fruit of tall herbaceous perennial plant, (*Elettaria cardamomum* Maton) belongs to the family *Zingiberaceae*. It is a shade loving plant cultivated at an altitude of 600 to 1200 m above MSL with an annual rainfall of 1500 to 4000 mm and a temperature range of 10 to 35°C. Till recently India was the main producer and exporter of cardamom. Of late Guatemala has emerged as a keen competitor to Indian cardamom in the international spice market. Tanzania, Sri Lanka, El Salvador, Vietnam, Laos, Cambodia and Papua New Guinea are the other cardamom growing countries. In India, cardamom is cultivated in the southern states of Kerala, Karnataka and Tamil Nadu. During

2006-07, Kerala accounts for 59% of the cultivation and production followed by 35% in Karnataka and 6% in Tamil Nadu.[1]

Origin

The genus *Elettaria* is one of the few compact and small natural groups of plants whose origin is evergreen rainforests of South India and Srilanka from where it spread to other tropical countries. From time immemorial, India is known as home of cardamom. Until 1800 the world's supply came from evergreen monsoon forests of the Western Ghats in South India and Sri Lanka. Cardamom was an article of Greek trade during 4th century B.C. It was listed among the Indian spices liable to duty at Alexandria in A.D. 176. Active cultivation of cardamom in India was taken up by the erstwhile Travancore Government in 1823 A.D. Cardamom cultivation in India is concentrated mostly in those regions, which form the natural habitat of spices except for a small area in North Kanara and adjoining southern districts in Karnataka and Wynad district in Kerala where it is grown as a subsidiary crop in arecanut gardens. It is also not uncommon to see its performance as a mixed crop with coffee in suitable packets. The present cardamom-growing tract in India is concentrated mainly in those regions, which forms natural habitat of the species.

It lies between $8^{0}30'$ and $14^{0}30'$ N latitude and longitude of 75-70'E. It is an elongated tract from North to South extending over 2000 Km, Sirsi of Karnataka to Thirunelveli of Tamil Nadu. East to West, it is a narrow belt of land distributed over the Western Ghats. The important areas of cultivation are Nelliampathy, Wynad and Idukki in Travancore Cochin (Malabar) region in Kerala state. Uttar Kannada, Shimoga, Hassan and Chickmagalur, hills of Kodagu (Coorg) districts in Karnataka; Northern and Southern foot hills of Nilgiris, Didigul, Theni, Salem and Tirunelveli and parts of Coimbatore districts in Tamil Nadu.

Chemistry of cardamom

The composition of cardamom varies with the seeds and the capsules and its volatile oil[2], as detailed below:

Seeds

Composition	Per cent
Moisture	7-10
Total ash	3.8-6.9
Water soluble ash	1.3-5.05
Crude fibre	6.7-12.8
Starch	39.0-49.9
Phosphorus	0.215
Calcium	0.3
Sodium	0.015
Potassium	1.2
Iron	0.012
Volatile oil	5.5-10.5
Alkalinity of ash	0.4-2.4
Acid insoluble ash	1.3-5.0
Crude protein	7.0-14.0
Vitamins (mg/100g)	
Vitamin A	175IU/100g
Vit B1 (thiamine)	0.18
Vit B2 (Riboflavin)	0.235
Vitamin C	12.0
Niacin	2.3

Capsules

Compounds	Per cent
Moisture	20.0
Carbohydrates	42.1
Protein	10.2
Ether extract	2.2
Mineral matter (total ash)	5.4
Calcium	0.13
Phosphorus	0.16
Iron	5 mg/100g
Volatile oil	7.4
Crude fibre	20.1

Flavor profile

The volatile oil is commercially extracted from the seeds, which varies from 6.6-10.6% in seeds of *Mysore* and *Malabar* types grown in India. However, the oil content is low in the immature capsules in the order of 4-5%, while it was 0.2% in the husk. The aroma differences in various sources of cardamom are attributed to the proportion of the esters and 1,8 cineole. The unique aroma of cardamom is contributed by a combination of two major compounds namely, α -terpinyl acetate and 1,8 - cineole. The *Malabar* and *Mysore* types differ in the composition of their volatile oils. The oil of *Malabar* type is more camphory in aroma owing to the higher content of 1,8-cineole, while *Mysore* type or "Alleppy green" is more of α-terpinyl acetate contributing to the mild spicy flavor.

Medicinal and Pharmacology

Medicinal properties

The major medicinal properties of cardamom essential oil are antiseptic, carminative, digestive, diuretic, stimulant, stomachic, tonic and anti-spasmodic, antimicrobial and anti-inflammatory activities. Powdered cardamom seeds are invariably mixed with ground ginger, cloves and caraway and used mainly for combating digestive ailments. It is used as a powerful pleasant aromatic stimulant, carminative, stomachic and diuretic. Use of cardamom checks nausea and vomiting. In the present day, cardamom is used invariably as cardiac stimulant and may prevent teeth cavities. The seeds are aromatic, acrid, sweet, cooling, stimulant, carminative, stomachic, diuretic, cardiotonic, abortifacient and are useful in bronchitis, hemorrhoids, stangury, renal and vesical calculi, anorexia, dyspepsia, gastropathy and vitiated condition of vata. The seed is fragrant tonic to the heart, stomachic, laxative, lessens inflammation, useful in headache.

Pharmacological properties

Cardamom has antimicrobial activity. Seeds have inhibitory effect against microbes. The terpenoid constituents are responsible for the antifungal and antibacterial effects. Cardamom oil is effective as an antioxidant for cotton seed oil. Cardamom oil is used for its uplifting and invigorating properties and helps in digestion and nausea. It is used as an aphrodisiac, helpful in countering the irritation experienced during premenstrual tension (PMS) and works well on the respiratory system, to ease coughs and warming the body. The volatile oil of cardamom seeds is more effective in inhibiting the growth of the microbial species examined than fixed oil and the inhibitory effect against some pathogenic fungi increased with increasing concentration of volatile oil and had highly inhibitory effect on the selected pathogenic bacteria. Moreover, it exhibits highly cytotoxic and anticarcinogenic activities against human tumour cell lines. Volatile oil of cardamom has a noticeable effect as anti-inflammatory agent. The volatile oil of cardamom can be a potential grain protectant by killing various life stages of the stored product insects attacking wheat through contact and fumigant action.

Uses

Cardamom seeds are widely used in Indian cooking for flavouring food and as carminative. It is an essential ingredient in garam masala and also used as a breath freshener. A Popular nasal application is prepared by using extracts of cardamom, neem and myrobalans along with animal fat and camphor. Cardamom seeds are chewed to prevent unpleasant smell in mouth, indigestion, nausea and vomiting due to sickness and to prevent pyrosis (excessive watering in mouth). Gargling with the infusion of cardamom and cinnamon is known to cure pharyngitis, sour throat, and hoarseness during the infective stage of flue. Powdered seeds of cardamom boiled with tea-water imparts very pleasant aroma to the tea and it can be used as medicine for scanty urination, diarrhea, decently, palpitation of the heart, exhaustion due to over work, depression etc. It is believed that eating cardamom capsule daily along with a tablespoon of honey improves eye site, strengthens the nervous system and thus improves health of the person. Cardamoms are capable of destroying Kapa and poison, promote skin complexion, destroy itching, pustules and akotha. Also used for asthma, burning sensation, cold and cough, diseases of bladder and kidney, flatulence, heart weakness, indigestion, scanty urine and piles.

Botany

Cardamom (*Elettaria cardamomum* Maton) belongs to the natural order Scitaminae under the family Zingiberaceae. The genus *Elettaria* consists of about six or seven species distributed in India, Sri Lanka, Malaysia and Indonesia; only *E. Cardamomum* is economically important.

It is herbaceous perennial (2-5 m in height) having underground (sub terrain) rhizomes with aerial pseudo stems (tillers) made of leaf sheaths. Studies on vegetative growth indicated that suckers continue their growth for a period of about 18 months from time of emergence. The rate of linear growth was maximum during June and July when the suckers have attained an age of about one year. The development of reproductive buds (panicles) was noticed in 89 per cent of them, indicating that the suckers require about 10 to 12 months to attain maturity. It takes almost 10 months for a vegetative bud to develop and about a year for the panicle to emerge from the newly formed tillers.

Inflorescence is a long panicle with racemose clusters arising from the underground stem, but coming up above the soil. Pattanshetty and Prasad[3] and Parameswar[4] have made detailed observations on panicle production, its growth, duration of flowering etc. The linear growth of the panicles extends over a period of about seven months. The rate of growth was maximum during April, it was slower both during the earlier and later stages. The growth habit of the panicles and the shape and size of the capsules vary in different cultivated varieties/types of cardamom. These panicle either grow erect (*Mysore*), prostrate (*Malabar*) or in a semi erect manner (*Vazhukka*). Multiple branching (compound panicle) of panicles appears in certain cultivars. In such case the central peduncle undergoes further branching of secondary and tertiary branches producing compound panicle types.

Flowers appear on the panicle after 4 months and flowering continues for a period of 6 months. The flowers are bisexual; bracts linear, oblong and persistent; racemose sepals 3; petals 3, unequal, lip longer with violet carpels 3; style 1; ovary – trilocular; axile placentation; ovules-numerous in each carpel. Normally, flowering in cardamom is seen throughout the year on panicles produced during the current as well as on panicles produced during the previous year. The peak flowering is spread over a period of six months in May to October. The time required from flower/bud initiation to full bloom stage ranges from 26 to 34 days. Capsule development takes about 110 to 120 days from the full bloom stage.[5]

The maximum numbers of flowers open during early hours of the day. Anthesis follows immediately. In Mudigere region of Karnataka, flowering commences at 3.30 AM and continued till 7.30 AM. The dehiscence of anthers takes place immediately followed by anthesis at 3.30 AM which continues up to 7.30 AM. The maximum pollen bursting occurs between 5.30 AM and 6.30 AM. The pollen grains are round, are mostly found in single and measure 87.6 μ on an average in diameter. By appearance 85.2 per cent of the pollen grains are fertile but germination a maximum of 70.1 per cent germinate on artificial medium containing 20 per cent sucrose and 1 per cent agar. Studies on viability of pollen grains indicate that only 6.5% of pollen grains remain viable after 2 hours of storage. After 6-8 hours of storage, the percentage of viability was practically zero.[5] Pollen fertility is maximum at full bloom stage and low at the beginning and end of flowering periods.[6] With respect to morphology, pollen of all the three varieties of cardamom are round in shape and the pollen mass appear as a creamy powder. The pollen grains of Mysore type are the largest and that of Vazhukka type the smallest.

Though cardamom has bisexual flowers and is self compatible, cross pollination is the rule. Self pollination is hindered in due to the slight protrusion of the stigma above the stamens. In cardamom, cross pollination is mediated by activity of the bees (*Apis cerana, Apis indica and Apis dorsata*) as pollinators. Cardamom flowers remain in bloom for 15-18 hours. Stigma receptivity and pollen viability are maximum during morning hours. The receptivity is maximum between 8 AM and 10 AM when 72% of the opened flowers set fruit. After 10 AM the stigma receptivity decreases gradually and only 24% of the flowers opening at 4 PM set fruit. It is reported that receptivity of stigma is highest between 8 AM and

12 noon.[5,7] Parvathi *et al.*[8] and Belavadi *et al.*[9] noticed that the peak receptivity around 12 noon and coincides with peak pollinator activity. The active foraging of bees is seen in the morning hours and is instrumental in increasing the fruit set in cardamom.

Pollination behaviour

In cardamom, pollination is effected by the activity of bees, two species namely *Apis cerena indica* F. (Indian hive bee) and *Apis dorsata* F. (Rock bee) constitute more than 95 percent of all the flower visitors and are the true pollinating agents. The active foraging of bees is seen in the morning hours of the day which help in increasing the fruit set of cardamom. Honeybees visit cardamom flowers during flowering season for collecting nectar and pollen and they do help in attaining over 90 per cent pollination.

The mean number of flowers open per day per plant is 34.5. The optimum bee visit for pollination is 3 to 5. In general, bee activity starts by around 7.30 a.m and continues till 6.30 in the evening, the peak is between 11.00 a.m to 1.00 p,m. On a clear day a flower is visited as many as 120 times, on a cloudy day 57 times and a rainy day 20 times on an average.[30]

The extent of fruit set recorded in different months indicates fruit set is high (50 to 59 per cent) during June, July, August and September because of high prevailing humidity. During the dry season from December to March, there was practically no fruit set. The fruit is globose or elipsoid, thin walled, smooth or with longitudinal ridges when ripe. The fruit colour is green and turn yellow on ripening. Seeds are white when unripe and turn to brown on ageing and become black on maturity and their numbers per capsule vary between 10-20 in different genotypes. Bee pollinated fruits were found to contain average of 10 seeds per capsule in South India, while it was 14 in Papua New Guinea.

Species and cultivars

Elettaria cardamomum Maton. is a small genus with 3-4 species in East and South- East Asia. The botanical identity of

Elettaria *cardamomum* Maton is no longer contentious; what is problematic is the vernacular name 'cardamom' for the spice, which is often also used for many other taxa, particularly *Amomum* species.

Two botanical varieties have been distinguished based on the size of the fruits, one for the wild taxon and one for the cultivated forms. They are

- *Elettaria cardamomum* var. *major* Thw. Comprising the 'wild' indigenous cardamom of Sri Lanka or Greater oblong cardamom or Long cardamom.
- *Elettaria cardamomum* var. *minor* Watt (syn. *Elettaria cardamomum* var. *minuscula* Burtkill) comprising all the cultivated groups. This cultivated cardamom can be grouped into many cultivar groups, the two most important ones being cv. Group Malabar and cv. Group Mysore.

In addition to the two main varieties, a few more have been recognised recently. All the varieties and races are interfertile and the observed variations are probably due to natural crossing. Based on the adaptability, nature of the panicle, shape and size of fruits three types of cultivated small cardamom *viz*., *Malabar*, *Mysore* and *Vazhukka* have been identified. Two more varieties mysorensis and laxiflora, have been recognized based on some morphological characters. The Sri Lankan wild cardamom is recognized as *Elettaria ensal* Abheywickrama.[10] Lot of confusion prevails over the botanical identity of Sri Lankan wild cardamom and the Indian cardamom varieties mentioned above. Various authors have named cardamom varieties differently.

Sri Lankan wild cardamom: *Elettaria ensal* Abheywickrama (*E. major* Thawaites)

Malaysian and Indonesian : *Elettaria longituba* (Ridl.)

Recently, Sakai and Nagamasu[11] while studying the Zingiberaceae of Indonesia listed seven species of *Elettaria* from the region (*E. rubida, E. stolonifera, E. kapitensis, E. surculosa, E. linearicrista, E. longipilosa* and *E. brachycallyx*).

Cytology

The chromosomal numbers are 2n=48 and 2n = 52. Cardamom is considered to be a balanced tetraploid. Allied genera such as *Globa, Balbifera, Phoemaria, Amomum sps* and *Alpinia sps* also possess 2n=48 and are considered to be evolved from a common basic number, x=12. The *Mysore* and *Malabar* varieties of cardamom possess 2n=50 and 2n=48 chromosomes, respectively and aneuploidy as well as structural alterations in the chromosome have contributed to the varietal differentiation.[12] Earlier workers have reported that cardamom is of amphidiploid origin from wild species and the two species considered to be the putative parents are the Sri Lankan cardamom *E. major* and the Malaysian species *E. longituba*.

Breeding and biotechnology

Genetic resources

In spite of its prominence in world trade from time immemorial, cardamom received research attention for genetic up gradation only in the second half of this century. Two surveys during 1950's were conducted in cardamom growing areas in India to record the genetic resources and wild populations and to understand the geographical distribution and environmental impact on cardamom. Six research organisations *viz*., Indian Institute of Spices Research (ICAR), Cardamom Research Centre, Appangala, Kodagu, Karnataka; Indian Cardamom Research Institute (ICRI), Myladumpara and its Regional Research Stations, Sakleshpur, Karnataka and Tadiyangudsi in Tamil Nadu; Regional Research Station, Mudigere (UAS, Bangalore); Cardamom Research Station, Pampadumpara (KAU, Kerala) are at present engaged in research for improvement of cardamom. Regular surveys are being undertaken by these institutions for gathering the variable germplasm and exploiting the desirable genes of these accessions through various crop improvement techniques. The collections of large number of indigenous lines are being conserved in different centers.

In situ conservation

In this method, accessions are maintained in field conditions itself as clonal repository or field or gene banks.

Ex situ conservation

Short term storage by inducing slow growth in micro propagated plants. Geetha *et al.*[13] and Nirmal Babu *et al.*[14] reported that of the various parameters tested, the best method of inducing slow growth was half-strength Ms medium without growth regulators, supplemented with 15 g/L each of sucrose and manitol in screw-capped culture tubes and incubation at 22±2°C with photoperiod of 12 h light/12 h dark and a light intensity of 2500 lux. Cultures maintained under these conditions can be conserved for one year without subculture. Conserved plantlets multiplied normally and were planted in soil with an 85% success rate.

Long term storage by means of cryopreservation using liquid nitrogen at 196°C. Cryopreservation of cardamom seeds in the vapour phase of liquid nitrogen has been reported by Chaudhary and Chandel.[15]

Characterization

Cardamom being a cross-pollinated crop, a lot of phenotypic variants exists in nature. Some of the exceptional variants have panicles of various types, terminal panicle, branched raceme, female sterility and cleistogamy. Krishnamurthy *et al.*[5] classified the germplasm accessions at the Regional Research Station, Mudigere and recognized 26 distinct types. A descriptor for cardamom was brought out during 1994 by the International Plant Genetic Resources Institute, Rome, Italy.[16]

Wide range of variations was observed between and with in cultivars of small cardamom for economically important characters. At the Cardamom research Centre of the Indian Institute of Spices Research in Kodagu district of Karnataka state, the clustering pattern of 310 cardamom accessions indicated that the possibilities of a common ancestral and close relationship of the genotypes of three groups (*Malabar*, *Mysore* and *Vazhukka*) from major cardamom growing regions. Accessions from same cultivar group scattered in different clusters.[17]

Genetic improvement

The major objectives of the crop improvement programme in cardamom are to develop clones having wider adaptability to different agro ecological conditions and also to evolve genotypes with high yield, superior capsule characters and resistance / tolerance to drought, major pest and diseases. Breeding methods such as selection, hybridization, mutation breeding, polyploidy breeding and tissue culture have been employed in cardamom.

Clonal selection

The improved varieties identified as far are evolved by selecting superior plants with desirable characters of higher yield and superior capsule characters from land race populations. The highly heterozygous nature of the crop and the ability to multiply selections by clonal propagations has contributed to this success. Selection is made '*in situ*' in planters field and forests the selected plants are multiplied clonally, subjected to preliminary evaluation and subsequently evaluated in comparative yield trial and multi location trial to confirm their superiority and adaptability. Selection of cardamom is highly location specific in their agro-ecological requirements. The improved selections are much superior to the local clones with regard to yield and capsule characters.[18] Salient features of varieties in vogue are summarized in *Table 1*.

Inter-varietal hybridization

Since cardamom is amenable to both sexual and vegetative propagation, hybridization is a very useful tool for crop improvement. Research at various Institutes has led to the isolation of high yielding recombinants and heterotic hybrids. The diallel cross combinations were more vigorous compared to the parental lines.[5] Hybrid vigour in seedlings of cardamom was observed with respect to plant height, number of leaves per plant, leaf length and breadth.[19] The hybrids, MHC 18, MHC 10 and MHC 12 had hybrid vigour with regard to yield and yield contributing characters.[20] Appreciable heterosis was recorded over standard parent for yield characters in desirable direction and identified high yielding mosaic resistant hybrids.[21] Genetic analysis of diallel hybrids revealed the influence of dominance and over dominance in the manifestation of quantitative characters.[22]

Polycross breeding

Since cardamom is a cross pollinated crop, polycross method of breeding is ideal to evolve superior types. Elite clones having predominantly desirable characters are planted together on isolated plot. Beehives are maintained in the plot for assured pollination so that maximum fruit set and high number of seeds per capsule can be obtained. Initial results on the impact of selection in a polycross progeny population for cardamom improvement are encouraging.

Inter-generic hybridization

Although a few improved high yielding varieties of cardamom have been evolved, combining yield and cardamom mosaic resistance has not been possible. To achieve this objective, intergeneric crosses were made using *Ammomum subulatum*, *Alpinia neutans*, *Hedychium flavascene* and *Hedychium coronarium* as male parents. A few fruits have been obtained only in the cross involving *Alpinia neutans*; in other crosses no seed was set.[23] The results of intergeneric crosses are not encouraging.[5,24] Compatibility barriers prevented the formation of fruits in these cross combinations.[24] Investigations are in progress to locate the causes of cross incompatibility.

Mutation breeding

For developing clones tolerant to cardamom mosaic (*katte*) virus and drought, seeds, rhizomes of cardamom have been subjected to X rays, Nitrosomethyl Urea (NMU), Diethyl Sulphate

ICRI 3	1993	Selection	Selection from Malabar type
ICRI 4	1997	Selection	Clonal selection from Vadagaraparai area of lower pullenys, a Malabar type
ICRI 5	2006	Hybridization	MCC260 X MCC 49
ICRI 6	2006	Selection	Clonal Selection
IISR Suvashini	1997	Selection	Clonal selection from OP progenies of Cl.37 Malabar type
IISR Avinash	1999	Selection	Clonal selection from OP progenies of CCS- Malabar type
IISR Vijetha	2001	Selection	Clonal selection from Natural katte escapes (NKE 12) Malabar type

Breeding for drought tolerance

The development of new varieties or cultivars with high yield and tolerance to drought condition is of prime importance in cardamom breeding. In recent years, emphasis has been given to survey problem areas for identifying drought escapes. Such collections made from different centers are under evaluation. Selection of cardamom genotypes were carried out using parameters such as relative water content, membrane leakage, stomatal resistance and specific leaf weight, and significant variations have been noted among cultivars.[31]

Gurumurthy *et al.*[32] screened the 12 elite cardamom clones for drought tolerance under the hill zone conditions of Karnataka. Under no irrigation and irrigation at 50% ASM, the performance of P-3 and P-6 was superior compared to other clones in terms of yield. Laboratory studies subjecting leaf discs to Sullivan's drought tolerance test have shown clone P-3 and CL-670 as having least leakage. Higher dry matter production of 350g/plant was recorded in clone P-6 followed by CL-664 (277g/plant). The clone P-6 maintained higher RWC and LAI during the stress. Cultivars Mysore and Vazhukka are susceptible to stress and Malabar is relatively tolerant to stress.[33] Screening of sixty seven genotypes for relative water content, specific leaf weight and number of stomata per microscopic field (60x) recorded significant variation between genotypes. Relative water content (per cent reduction over control) ranged from 11.5-27.12 per cent with a mean of 21.49 per cent. Specific leaf weight was ranged from 4.07 -6.7 mgcm^2 with a mean of 5.25 mgcm^2. Number of stomata per microscopic field (60x) ranged from 6.5-17.75 with a mean of 12.99. Genotypes RR1, Cl 893 and LR1 are found to relatively tolerant to moisture stress. They maintained relatively high biomass under stress compared to NKE-12, NKE-9 and RR2.[34]

Breeding for quality

The most commercially desirable item in cardamom is its volatile oil. The oil content in cardamom varies from 5.5 to 8.7 per cent. The major chemical constituents which impart sweet flavour to the oil are terpinyl acetate, linalyl acetate, linalool etc. '*Mysore*' possesses more terpinyl acetate compared to '*Malabar*' while the later possesses more 1,8-cineole which impart harsh camphory note to the oil.[35] Evaluation of thirty-three germplasm has also led to the identification of two accessions (Acc.221 and Acc.223), which contained 7.8 % essential oil content consistently for three years. Its oil had high concentration of aroma bearing constituents of ethers such as alpha terpinyl and linalyl acetate and low concentration of 1,8-cineole.[36]

Biotechnology

Micropropagation

Cardamom is one of the first crops where commercialization of micropropagation has been achieved. It is being cross-pollinated crop, clones are ideal for generating true to type planting material from high yielding clones. *'Katte'* disease caused by virus is one of the major production constraints in cardamom. Production of virus-free planting material is considered to be the most important input in disease management program and to check disease spread. High rate of multiplication coupled with additional advantage of obtaining uniform and disease free planting material makes micropropagation a preferred method over the conventional method.

Micropropagation technique for cardamom has been standardized.[37,38,39,40,41] Its further refinement through increased axillary branch multiplication reported by Vatsya *et al.*[42] Priyadarshan *et al.*[43] and Anon.[44]

Plant regeneration from callus and production of somaclones

Rao *et al.*[37] reported successful regeneration of plantlets from callus culture of seedling explants in cardamom. Plantlet formation via adventitious shoots from callus cultures was reported by Priyadharshan and Zachariah.[45] Protocols for organogenesis and plant regeneration from rhizome and vegetative bud-derived callus cultures have also been standardized at the Indian Institute of Spices Research, Calicut, Kerala.[46] This regeneration system (with 20-50 plantlets per culture) is being used at present for large scale production of somaclones and selection of useful genotypes there from. High amount of variability was noticed among the somaclones for morphological characters in the culture vessels itself.

Propagation through enhanced axillary branching method

The MS medium fortified with IAA, BAP, Kinetin, calcium pantothenate, biotin and coconut water has given the best results using shoot primordial as explants.[43] Reghunath and Bajaj[47] have outlined the culture method, using shoot and inflorescence primordium explants. The number of axillary branches was highest in medium containing 4mg/l BAP and 0.5 mg/l NAA and it was enhanced by coconut water.

In vitro rooting

The excised axillary shoots can be rooted on a semi-solid medium of half strength MS salt and 0.5 percent activated charcoal for 1 week, followed by sub culturing in ½ MS medium containing 1.5 m/l IBA. Rooted shoots were transferred to ½ MS liquid medium containing only mineral salts and then shifted to green house for hardening. For planting, vermiculite:fine sand (1:1) was found the best giving 92 percent establishment.[47]

Evaluation of tissue culture plants

The results showed that the tissue culture plants of well-managed estates gave 25 -- 36 per cent increase in yield over seedlings.[48] Lukose *et al.*[41] carried out first, statistically laid out trial to evaluate the performance of TC plants together with suckers and seedlings and reported non significant variations among TC plants. Sudharshan *et al.*[49] reported the results of large scale evaluation with an overall variability of 4.5 per cent in tissue cultured plants as against 3.0 per cent in open pollinated seedling progeny for the given set of characters. Reghunath and Priyadarshan[50] while studying four lines of plantlets regenerated from axenic culture of juvenile shoot primordial reported considerable variation of 13.67 per cent for panicle branching pattern and plant height.

Nursery management

Cardamom is propagated either through seeds or vegetative means and being a cross-pollinated crop the seedling population is not uniform. Only 35 per cent of the plants are good yielders in a plantation raised from seedling population.[5] Hence, vegetative propagation is normally adopted for multiplication of elite clones. Vegetative propagation can be either through suckers or tissue culture.

The seeds can be collected from any elite plantation from fully ripe capsules preferably from second to third round of harvest in September and are then either washed in water and sown immediately or mixed with wood ash and dried for 2 to 9 days in room temperature. Storage of seeds results in loss of viability and delay in germination. Immediate sowing resulted in maximum germination. Germination was highest when sown in September. Gradual decline in germination was observed when sown on 1st August, 15th August, 30th August, 14th September, 29th September and 14th October, respectively. Cardamom seeds sown immediately after harvest (September) germinate uniformly, and seedlings are ready for transplanting at the end of 10 months. The ideal sowing season has been reported to be November - January for Kerala and Tamil Nadu and September for Karnataka.

Germination is significantly correlated with maximum and minimum temperature prevalent in the area as the seeds fail to germinate at temperature less than 15°C and greater than 35°C. Germination will optimum at 30°C (70.9-73.0% RH) with the highest percentage during September-October. The normal light requirement for cardamom nursery was found to be 55 per cent optimum for better growth and development of seedlings in the nursery. Mulching of seedbeds influence the germination of seeds. Mulching with coir dust, paddy straw and dry sal leaves enhances the germination.

Seedlings of four to five leaf stages from the primary nursery beds are generally transplanted in the secondary nursery at a distance of 20 to 25cm or in polythene bags (20 x 20 cm). In Karnataka, where seeds are sown during August - September, transplanting in the secondary nursery is done during November - January. In Kerala and Tamil Nadu, seedlings from primary beds are transplanted to secondary nursery beds at a spacing of 20 x 20 cm during June-July and the rate of mortality can be minimized by transplanting at the four-five leaf stage.[51]

Seed treatment with *Trichoderma* culture (50 ml spore suspension for 100 g of seed) is desirable as a prophylactic measure for managing nursery rot diseases. At the time of preparation of beds, incorporation of VAM multiplied in recommended organic medium is to be incorporated. For raising polybag seedlings (preferably bio-degradable polybags), potting mixture may be prepared by using 3:1:1 soil rich in organic matter, well rotten cow dung or vermicompost and sand. VAM and *Trichoderma* can also be added to the potting mixture (250 g mixed with 25 kg of well rotten cow dung). If growth of the seedlings is not adequate, spraying vermiwash once in a month is desirable (20 ml per plant). The diseases in the nurseries may be managed by regular surveillance and adopting phytosanitary measures. Restricted application of Bordeaux mixture 1% may be taken up to control rot disease at the initial stage itself. Changing the nursery site is benefited to ward off pests and diseases and for vigorous growth of seedlings.[52]

Suckers from elite clones can be used for establishing plantations capable of high productivity. Plants raised from suckers come to bearing earlier than seedlings. Suckers should not be used in areas where katte and other virus diseases (such as *Kokke kandu* and Niligiri necrosis) are common.

Planting and aftercare

Site selection and shade requirement

The shade canopy provides suitable environment by maintaining humidity and evaporation at suitable level and shade requirements vary from place to place and depend on the lay of land, soil type, rainfall pattern and crop combination etc. Cardamom yield level was high under 65-70 per cent light intensity and total biomass, chlorophyll and protein contents, photochemical activity gets adversely affected when grown under full light (100 per cent), when compared to medium light (45-55 per cent). Forty percent reduction in growth of plants exposed to full light was observed compared to those exposed to medium light. Laboratory studies on photosynthetic efficiency in cardamom indicated that efficiency was greater under low light intensities (30 to 107 micro Einstein per sec per sq meter) than at higher ones.

Preparation of main field

Cardamom is generally cultivated in forest area with an overhead umbrella canopy to get filtered shade. If land is sloppy, it is advisable to start cleaning from the top and work down wards. In sloppy areas, adequate soil and water conservation measures are necessary while preparing the land for planting. Planting in trenches across the slopes in low rainfall areas, diagonal planting and mulching the soil will help in soil and water conservation.

Spacing

Spacing should be decided based on variety and duration of crop in the field. '*Mysore*' and '*Vazhukka*' types are vigorous and need wider spacing. '*Malabar*' types need closer spacing as comparatively smaller plants.

Higher yield in cardamom seedlings planted at 2 x 1m in hill slopes and 2.1 x 2.1m in flat lands was reported in Karnataka. The trench method of planting with a spacing of 2 x 1 m results in better growth and yield. In general, '*Mysore*' and '*Vazhukka*' types planted at a spacing of 3 x 3 m or 2.4 x 2.4m in high rainfall or irrigated areas. A spacing of 1.8 x1.8 m or 2 x 2 m is suitable for cardamom growing areas of Karnataka. .

Method of planting

The trench method of planting (60 x 30 cm) with a spacing of 2 x 1 m results in the best growth and yield with a greater moisture retention than the pit system of planting. '*Mysore*' and '*Vazhukka*' types, usually planted in the pits of 90 x 90 x 45 or 90 cm, where as, 45 x 45 x 45 cm pits are generally opened during April-May after pre-monsoon showers are used for planting '*Malabar*' types. Pits are filled with mixture of topsoil and compost or well rotten farmyard manure and 40 g of rock phosphate.

Planting season

Planting season is decided based on topography and rainfall pattern. Normally planting is done in June-July. In areas experiencing heavy south-west monsoon, planting is either completed before July or is taken up in August-September, so as to avoid heavy rains in July. Early planting gives better establishment and growth than late plantings. Planting in low laying areas (such as valleys) should be done only after heavy rains by July. Better establishment and growth of seedlings were recorded in August planting in Mudigere of Karnataka. Cardamom suckers are planted from June to August on the surface or 15-20 cm deep below the surface. During the month of planting, minimum of 320 mm rainfall along with temperature range of 15.5 - 17.5°C (minimum) and 19.5 - 25.0°C (maximum) is required for better establishment.

Planting

Ten or eighteen month old cardamom seedlings are planted in pits by taking small portion of filled soil and adding rock phosphate

(40 g) in the centre of pit and seedling is placed in the centre of depression. Soil is then replaced taking care that the roots are distributed in their normal position and well pressed around the base of the clump. Planting need to be done just above the ground level to avoid rotting in heavy rains. Seedlings are normally planted in a pit at acute angle for promoting shoot production. In eighteen months old seedlings light root pruning need to be taken up. In case planting suckers, suckers may be placed in the slanting position and cover the base of rhizome with soil. After planting, cross-staking need to given immediately after planting to avoid damage due to wind. After transplanting, care should be taken to offset the transplanting shock and to save the seedlings from heavy rains.

Mulching

Mulch the plant base to reduce evapo transpiration and rain damages. Fallon leaves of the shade trees can be utilized for mulching. Sufficient mulch should be applied during November - December to reduce the ill effect of drought which prevails for nearly 4-5 months during summer. De-mulching is also equally important during May after the pre monsoon showers for facilitating honey bee movement to obtain better pollination and capsule setting and also provide better aeration and minimizes incidence of clump rot or rhizome rot. The practice of uncovering the panicles shortly after the commencement of flowering improves fruit set in cardamom.

Weeding and trashing

Clean weeding is to be limited to the plant bases (50 cm) and the inter rows are to be maintained by slash weeding. The weeded materials can be used for mulching. Trashed materials and fallen leaves may also used for mulching. Trashing the dry leaves, leaf sheaths and removal of yielded old suckers along with rhizomes may be carried out once in a year about a month after completion of final harvest, which can be used, for composting. Trashing thrice a year and cleaning the plant bases during monsoon months helps in better pollination, elimination of breeding sites of sucking pests and reduce rhizome rot incidence.

Irrigation management

Cardamom is generally grown as a rainfed crop and cardamom tracts of India experience a dry spell of about 5-6 months. Increased denudation of forests, deterioration in forest ecology, coupled with erratic trends of rainfall, leads to aridity effects, which adversely affect cardamom production. Since the roots of cardamom are shallow, moisture at the root zone does not last long and hence it is essential to irrigate the crop during January to May. Irrigation at 75 per cent available soil moisture (ASM) recorded favourable growth parameters compared to 25 per cent. Further, it was reported that, higher level of irrigation produced maximum capsules and capsule weight compared to irrigation at lower levels.

Cardamom irrigated at 25 per cent ASM and 75 per cent ASM produced 2.01 and 2.14 times more capsules than those without irrigation. Irrigation at 75 per cent ASM combined with high light resulted in the highest yield of 2618 kg/ha. Sprinkler irrigation equivalent to 4 cm rainfall at every 12-15 days would be quite sufficient for cardamom crop. Drip irrigation daily @8 liters/plant from January 15th onwards recorded significantly higher yield and this was followed by sprinkler irrigation once in 12 days. In low to medium rainfall areas (1200 to 2000mm), trench system of planting was found to conserve soil moisture. In areas having more than 7 per cent slope, of all along the contour, bench terracing of about 5-6 feet width has to be created for taking up cardamom planting. Agronomical practices like shade regulation, trench, terrace system of planting, provision of shelter belts, mulching, earthing up, vegetative barriers and intercropping help in better growth and development of cardamom besides effective soil and water conservation measures.

Drainage

Although cardamom requires high moisture level, it is very sensitive to high water table and consequent waterlogged situations. Drains should be opened at regular intervals so as to keep water table 30 cm below the ground surface for better growth. In valleys and high rainfall areas with medium slopes, suitable drains (45 cm depth and 30 cm width) have to be provided while planting in between two rows of cardamom. These drains have to be cleaned regularly to avoid stagnation of water during rainy season. This will also avoid rhizome and root rot to considerable extent.

Shade regulation

Shade requirement studies indicated that cardamom does not tolerate direct sunlight at the same time too much shade affects metabolic activities of plants. Hence, removal of excess shade is also essential so as to allow sufficient penetration. Shade has to be regulated based on the topography of land, moisture content etc. so as to get about 50 per cent filtered sunlight for proper growth and flowering. It should be done during summer (March-April) in the new planting areas and during May-June after the receipt of summer showers in the existing plantation. It is desirable to maintain a mixed population of medium sized shade trees, that facilitate shade regulation and to maintain more or less optimum conditions throughout the year. Balangi (*Artocarpus fraxinifolius* Wt), Nili (*Bisochofia javanica* Blum), Jack (*Artocarpus heterophyllus* Lamk), Red cedar (*Cedrela toona* Roxb), Karimaram (*Diospyros ebenum* Koenig), Karna (*Vernonia monocis* C.B. Darke), Nandi (*Lagerstroemia lanceolata*) and Spanish cherry (*Mimusops elengi*) are desirable as shade trees for cardamom. Cardamom grown under *Diospyros ebenum*, yielded 40-50 per cent higher than those planted under Jack, Nandi and Spanish cherry. Inclusion of black pepper, coffee and arecanut cardamom plantations adopting mixed cropping systems in Kerala and Karnataka was highly remunerative giving higher cost benefit ratios.

Trees having desirable characters such as leguminous species, defoliation during rainy season, self pruning habit, flowering during summer and medicinal value may be considered. Restricted loppings and leaf litter may be used for green leaf manuring or composting and recycling. Dinesh Kumar and Babitha[53] studied the rate of leaf fall from some common shade trees present in cardamom production system and characterized the same based on major nutrients. Most shade trees shed their leaves during September to December. Highest leaf shed was noticed in *Syzygium cumini*, followed by *Terminalia arjuna*. As far as major nutrients concerned, *Erythrina indica* was recorded higher contents of nitrogen and phosphorous, while *Lagerstroemia lanceolata* contained more potassium.

Pollination management

The number of honeybee colonies required for effective pollination of cardamom is minimum of four colonies (about 5000 foragers per colony) per hectare (3000 plants). In cardamom, by maintaining the beehives 9 to 13 percent increased yield were reported.

- Mulching during flowering period hinders bee pollination resulted in 33 to 44 per cent reduction in fruit set. Thus, demulching after the pre monsoon showers to facilitate better honey bee movement and capsule setting
- Bee pollination resulted in better quality capsules of uniform size and shape.
- Promoting use of beekeeping for pollination of cash crops will be of benefit to both the beekeeper who will receive money for the pollination services of his honeybees and harvest honey and to the farmer whose income will be increased through boosting crop productivity as a result of pollination services of bees.

Nutrient management

Manuring

Cardamom is generally grown in the rich fertile soils of the forest eco-system. Being a perennial crop sucker production is throughout the year and initiation of panicles and development of capsules spread over a period of eight to nine months in a year. As steady absorption and utilization of plant nutrients take place throughout the life cycle of cardamom, a regular application of nutrients should be followed for higher yields. Application of compost or farm yard manure @ 5 kg/plant/year in May-June is recommended. Application of 3-4 t of well rotten cattle or sheep manure apart from 30 kg each of N, P_20_5 and 40 kgs K_2O/acre greatly enhanced the yield in cardamom.[54] Thimmarayappa *et al.*[55] reported that integrated nutrient management with 25% organic manure + 75 % inorganic fertilizers and 50 % organic manure + 50 % inorganic fertilizers also recorded yields at par with 75 % organic manure + 25 % inorganic fertilizers. Application of recommended NPK nutrients as organic fertilizers (50 per cent each as FYM and neem cake + 50 per cent P each as bone meal and rock phosphate + 50 per cent K as wood ash) is effective in increasing the yield and quality of cardamom.[56]

Application of organic manures such as neem cake @ 1 kg or poultry manure/farmyard manure/compost/vermicompost @ 2kg per plant is recommended once in a year during May-June. Mussorie rock phosphate or bone meal may be applied based on soil analysis. As majority (nearly 70 per cent) of cardamom roots were confined to shallow depth of 5 - 40 cm and 30 - 50 cm radius and being a surface feeder, manures and fertilizers should be applied at a radius within 50 cm.

Bio fertilizers

Three species of vesicular arbuscular mycorrhizal (VAM) fungi (*Glomus macrocarpum*, *G. fasciculatum* and *Gigaspora coralloidea*) were recorded in the roots of cardamom plants. Per cent colonization in roots varied from 40 – 100 per cent in pre-monsoon samples and 63 - 94 per cent in post-monsoon samples. Seedlings inoculated with the VAM fungi grew taller, had more leaves and tillers, and greater seedling biomass and uptake of nutrients than control seedlings. Among the various mycorrhizal fungi tested, seedlings inoculated with *Gigaspora margarita* and *Glomus monosporum* exhibited significantly greater growth with increased uptake of nutrients.

Harvest

Cardamom suckers or seedlings start bearing after two years of planting. Panicles appear from the base of plant from January onwards and the flowering is from April to December, which may extend further. Peak flowering is observed during June to August and fruits mature in about 120 days after flowering. Fruits have trilocular capsules containing 15-20 seeds and on maturity seed turn black in colour.

Due to staggered and prolonged flowering, cardamom capsules mature and ready for harvesting successively at 10 – 15 days intervals over an extended period of 8 months (August to March). Generally harvesting is carried out at an interval of 15-30 days and completed in 8-9 rounds. Fruits (capsules) that are fully matured and retaining dark green colour of rind (peel) with black coloured seeds are ready for harvesting. Harvesting at over ripe stage leads to loss of green colour and capsule splitting during curing. Per cent recovery of dry capsules varies from 20-24 % in ripe capsules, 18-20 % in physiologically mature stage and 14-16 % in immature stage. Hence it is ideal to harvest cardamom at physiologically mature stage (green colour rind and black colour seeds). After harvesting, the freshly harvested capsules are cleaned and cured to reduce the moisture content from 80 % to 8-12 % in an optimum environment for retaining green colour to the maximum extent.

References

1. Anonymous, Area and production statistics of arecanut and spices. Directorate of Arecanut and Spices Development, Ministry of Agriculture, Government of India, Calicut, Kerala (2008).
2. J.S. Pruthi. Spices and Contiments. National Book Trust, New Delhi, India. (1987).
3. H.V. Pattanshetty and A.B.N. Prasad, Blossom biology, pollination and fruit set in cardamom. In: Proc. Intern. Sym. Subtropical and Tropical Horticulture (Vol I), Today and Tomorrow's Publishers, New Delhi, pp. 262-268 (1976).
4. N.S. Parameswar, Mysore *J. Agric. Sci.*, 7(2):205-213 (1973).
5. K. Krishnamurthy, M.M. Khan, K.K. Avadhani, J. Venkatesh, A.L. Siddaramaiah, A.K. Chakravarthy, and B.R Gurumurthy, Three decades of Cardamom Research at Regional Research Station, Mudigere, UAS, Bangalore 97 (1989).
6. R. Venugopal and N.S. Parameswar, Mysore *J. Agric Sci.*, **8**, 203-205 (1974).
7. K.M. Kuruvilla and K.J. Madhusoodanan, Spice India, **1**(6): 19-21 (1988).
8. C. Parvathi, Y.G. Shadakshari, V.V. Belavadi and H.M. Chandrappa, In: Pollination in tropics (G.K. Veeresh, R. Umashanker and K.N. Ganesan. eds), IUSSI, Bangalore, pp. 99-103 (1993).
9. V.V. Belavadi, C. Parvathi and B. Raju, *Recent Advances in Plantations Crop Research*, 318-322 (2000).
10. K.J. Madhusoodanan, K. Pradip Kumar and P.N. Ravindran. In: Cardamom, the genus *Elettraia* (Ravindran, P.N and K.J. Madhusoodanan, eds). Taylor and Francis, London, pp. 11-68 (2002).
11. S. Sakai and H. Nagamasu, *Edinb.J.Bot.*, **57**, 227-243 (2000).
12. R. Chandrasekhar and K. Sampathkumar, *J. Cytol and Genet.* **21**(1-2): 90-97 (1986).
13. S.P. Geetha, C. Manjula, and A. Sajina, *In vitro* conservation of genetic resources of spices. In: Proc. Kerala, Sci. Congress, Palakkad pp.12-16 (1995).
14. K. Nirmal Babu, S.P. Geetha, D. Minoo, P.N. Ravindran and K.V. Peter, *Plant Genetic Resources News Letter*. **119**:41-45 (1999).
15. R. Chaudhury and K.P.S. Chandel, *Seed Sci. Technol* **23**:235-240 (1995).

16. IPGRI. Descriptor for cardamom (*Elettaria cardamomum* Maton.).International Plant Genetic Resources Institute, Rome, pp 27-41 (1994).

17. D. Prasath and M.N. Venugopal *Plant Genetic Resources Newsletter*. **138**: 55-60 (2004).

18. M.N. Venugopal and D. Prasath. Green Technology. **5**: 14-17 (2003).

19. K. Padmini, M.N. Venugopal and S.J. Ankegowda *J. Spices and Aromatic Crops*. **9** (2):145-151 (2001).

20. K. Pradipkumar, K.M. Kuruvilla and K.J. Madhusoodanan, Hybrid vigour in cardamom. In: Proceedings XIV Plantation Crops Research Symposium (P. Rethinam, H.H. Khan, V.M. Reddy, P.K. Mandal and K. Suresh, eds) pp 78-80 (2002).

21. D. Prasath, M.N. Venugopal, R. Senthikumar and N.K. Leela, Euphytica **168**: 49-60.

22. D. Prasath and M.N. Venugopal, *Indian J. Genetics and Plant breeding*. **62** (2): 179-180 (2002).

23. N.S. Parameshwar, *Curr. Res.* **6**:10 (1997).

24. K.J. Madhusoodanan, K.M. Kuruvilla, P.M. Priyadarshan, and V.V. Radhakrishnan, Small cardamom - Botany and crop improvement. Cardamom Production - Technology, ICRI (Spices Board) 7-13 (1990).

25. ICRI Annual Report *1987*, Indian Cardamom Research Institute, Myladumpara, Idukki, Kerala (1987).

26. M.R. Sudharsan, *J. Plantation Crops*. **16**:365-369 (1989).

27. G. Subbarao, and R. Naidu, Breeding cardamom for 'Katte' disease resistance. In: Proc. Plantation Crops Research Symposium IV, Indian Society for Plantation Crops, Kasargod, Kerala, India, pp 320-324 (1985).

28. M.N. Venugopal, *J. Spices and Aromatic Crops* **8**(2):145-151 (1999).

29. M.N. Venugopal, M.J. Mathew, M. Anandaraj, *J Spices and Aromatic Crops* **8**(2):189-191 (1999).

30. M.N. Venugopal, D. Prasath and Ravindra Mulge, *J. Spices and Aromatic Crops.* **15**(1): 14 – 18 (2006).

31. IISR Annual Report 1996-1997, Indian Institute of Spices Research, Calicut, Kerala, India (1997).

32. B.R. Gurumurthy, H.M. Chandrappa, C Parvathi, B. Raju and S.M. Shanthaveerabhadraiah, In: Proceedings of the National seminar on

drought management in plantation crops (K.V. Satheesan, eds), Kottayam, Kerala, pp 25-29 (1996).

33. S.J. Ankegowda and K.S. Krishnamurthy, Response of cardamom ecotypes to moisture stress. In: Abstracts, Nat. Sem. Recent Advances in Plant Physiology, An inter-disciplinary approach to unravel plant functions, Central Plantation Crops Research Institute, Kasargod, Kerala, pp.54 (2000).

34. S.J. Ankegowda and K.S. Krishnamurthy, Screening of small cardamom cultivars for drought tolerance. In: Abstracts, Nat. Sem. Improving Crop Productivity in an Ecofriendly Environment: Physiological and Molecular Approaches, G.B Pant University of Agriculture and Technology, Pantnagar, pp.61 (2003).

35. S.J. Sarathkumara, E.V. Paciasothy and E.R. Jansz. *J. Science Food and Agriculture,* **36**(6): 491-198 (1985).

36. T.J. Zachariah, Ravidra Mulge and M.N. Venugopal, Quality of cardamom from different accessions. Developments in plantation crops research, pp337-340 (1998).

37. S.N.K. Rao, S. Narayanaswamy, E.K. Chacko and R. Doraiswamy, *Proc. Indian Academy of Sci. (Plant Sci.)*, **91**:37-41 (1982).

38. R. Nadgauda, A.F. Mascarenhas and K.J. *J. Plantation Crops*, **11**:60-64 (1983).

39. K.B. Kumar, Prakash Kumar, S.M. Balachandran, and R.D. Iyer, *J. Plantation Crops*, **13**:31-34 (1985).

40. Y.S. Rao, K. Mary Mathew, K. Pradikumar, K.J. Madhusoodanan, S.N. Potty and G.K. George, In: A manual on micropropagation of selected spices, Spices Board, Cochin pp 59 (1999).

41. R. Lukose, K.V. Saji, M.N. Venugopal and V.S. Korikanthimath, *Indian J Agri.Sci.*, **63**: 417-418 (1993).

42. B. Vatsya, K. Duiesh, A.R. Kundapurkar and S. Bhaskaran, *Plant Phy. Biochem.*, 14, 14-19 (1987).

43. P.M. Priyadarshan, K.M. Kuruvilla, K.J. Madhusoodanan and R. Naidu, New Trends in Biotechnology (N.S. Subba Rao, C. Rajagopalan and S.V. Ramakrishna, eds) Oxford IBH Publications, New Delhi, pp. 109-117 (1992).

44. Anonymous, Practical manual for handling cardamom tissue Cultured: ICRI, Spices Board, India p 37 (1992).

45. P.M. Priyadarsan and P.K. Zachariah, Studies on *in vitro* culture on cardamom (*Elettaria cardamomum* Maton)- Progress and

Limitations. In: Somers *et al* (Eds) VI International Congress on Plant Tissue and Cell Culture, Minneapolis, Minn. P. 107 (1986).

46. K. Nirmal Babu, J. Rema, R. Lukose, P.N. Ravindran, K. Johnson George, B. Sasikumar and K.V. Peter, Spices Biotechnology at NRCS, Calicut (Tech. Report), pp 11 (1993).

47. B.R. Reghunath, and Y.P.S. Bajaj, Biotechnology in Agriculture and Forestry Vol.19, Springer Verlag, Berlin, pp. 175-198 (1992).

48. Anonymous, Tissue Cultured Cardamom: Product Plan, Final Report, Spices Board, India (1996).

49. M.R. Sudharsan, S.K. Bhat and M. Narayanaswamy, Variability in tissue cultured cardamom plants. Proc. of National seminar on Biotechnology of Spices and Aromatic Crops, Calicut. pp 98-101 (1997).

50. B.R. Reghunath, and P.M. Priyadarshan, *Acta Horticulture*, 330: 235-242 (1993).

51. S.J. Ankegowda, Optimum leaf stage for transplanting small cardamom seedlings from primary nursery to secondary nursery. In: Abstracts of National Seminar on Physiological Interventions for Improved Crop Productivity and Quality: Opportunities and Constraints, December 12-14, 2003, S.V. College, Tirupati, pp.184 (2003).

52. Anonymous, Concepts, Principles, Basic standards, Production guidelines, Documentation, Inspection and Certification. In: Production of Organic Spices. Spices Board, Cochin (1998).

53. M. Dinesh Kumar and J. Babitha, *J. Spices and Aromatic Crops*, **15**(2): 108-114 (2006).

54. K.G. Shanmugavelu and V.N. Madhava Rao, Spices and Plantation crops, Popular Book Depot, Madras (1977).

55. M. Thimmarayappa, K.T. Shivashankar and S.M. Shanthaveerabhadraiah, *J. Spices and Aromatic Crops,* **9**: 57-59 (2000).

56. A.K. Sadanandan and S. Hamza, Effect of organic farming on soil quality, nutrient uptake, yield and quality of Indian spice, In: Abstracts of 18 th world congress of soil science, July 9-15, 2006, Philadelphia, USA (2006).

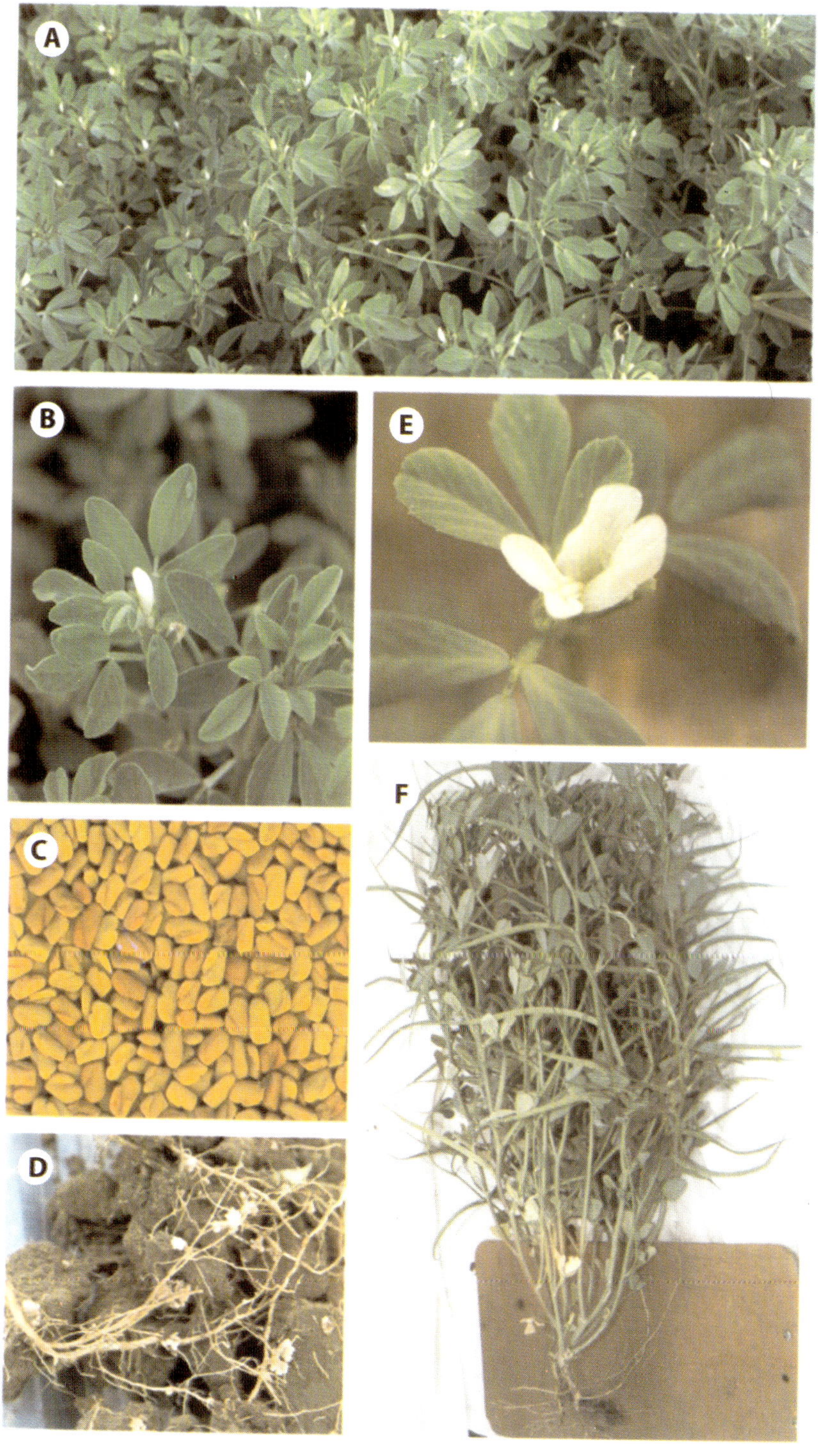
A
B
E
C
F
D

Figure 1. A. Fenugreek growing under dryland conditions of western Canada; B. A fenugreek flower in close up; C. Golden brown seeds of fenugreek grown in western Canada; D. Root of fenugreek plants with conspicuous root nodules; E. Close up of the papilionaceous corolla of self-pollinating fenugreek flower; and F. Entire fenugreek plant with trifoliate foliage bearing single and double pods.

powdered food color product comercialized under the name of '*fenugreek herb*' prepared from grounded leafy stems of fenugreek to give a green color to steamed pastry.[2] In India and China, the seeds are also used as a source of a food coloring dye and industrial mucilage. Fenugreek seed constitutes an essential part of Bengali five spice mixture- *panch foron*; Georgian spice mixture- *khmeli suneli*; Ethiopian spice mixture- *berbere*; Bulgarian spice mixture- *sharena sol.*[5]

Fenugreek is a novel crop for western Canadian prairie conditions[6] "Tristar" is the first North American fenugreek forage cultivar released by Lethbridge Research Center, Agriculture and Agri-Food Canada.[6] Fenugreek has several agro-ecological benefits for a number of reasons. It is an annual legume crop fixing atmospheric nitrogen and hence reduces the need for application of nitrogen fertilizers, thereby considerably reducing the production costs and is used effectively in short term rotations.[1] Less application of nitrogen fertilizers also reduces the possibility of contamination of water resources and hence fenugreek cultivation indirectly helps in conserving and protecting the natural environment.[1] Fenugreek is a dryland (rain-fed) crop which grows well under minimum irrigation.[4] In addition, it yields high quantity and high quality forage, is grown for hay or silage, does not cause bloat in cattle, and contains animal growth promoting substances (diosgenin) not reported in other forage legume species.[2]

Fenugreek improvement

The plant body is erect or prostrate, often bushy, having circular to slightly quadrangular greenish stems with purplish tinge bearing simple, trifoliate, stipulate leaflets and strongly branching tap root system bearing nitrogen-fixing root nodules. Fenugreek is a self-pollinating plant with small, white flowers (yellow when young) having papilionaceous corolla. The plants produce single or double pods bearing seeds at each nodule. The seed is rectangular to oval in shape and varies in colour from pale brown to golden yellow (Figure 1). Most species are diploids ($2n = 16$) (Petropoulos[3]);

however, it was reported that the haploid chromosome number (n) of *Trigonella* can also be 8, 9, 11 or 14.[7]

Optimal crop productivity for the crop in India has been obtained by planting crops in early October or November with 20-30 cms spacings, early sowing dates and forage cutting practices and application of minor irrigation.[2] According to Rosengarten[8] properly drained loamy soils characterised by pH ~ 8-8.5 is good for the crop growth. Judicious use of fertilizers, both organic and inorganic (such as nitrogen and phosphorus) and manures have been reported to be efficient in increasing the yield of fenugreek in India.[9] The use of wheat straw and some specific fungal species have also been reported to promote rate and efficiency of nodulation in fenugreek under salinity affected soil regimes.[10] Our research indicated that for high seed yield the optimal rate of phosphate application varied between 40-50 kg/ha; whereas, for optimal forage yield the phosphate application rate was between 50-60 kg/ha for the dark brown soil zones of the Canadian prairies.[11] We also found that combining the seed following swathing produced more seed in case of Tristar fenugreek in comparison to direct combining applications.[11] Foliar spray with growth regulators and different salts have been found effective in improving forage and seed yield as well as chemical constituents in fenugreek and other legumes.[12] Application of gibberellic acid (GA_3) has been found significantly efficient on the growth, maturity duration and seed yield of fenugreek under greenhouse condition. In our study, we came across that GA_3 application after post pod emergence period produced best seed yield. Additionally, our study reveals, spraying with ferrous sulphate, calcium chloride, cupric sulphate, magnesium sulphate and ammonium molybdate can bring improvement on seed yield and reduce maturation duration of fenugreek under greenhouse condition, whereas under field conditions those chemicals only have efficacy to reduce maturation duration.[13]

The different genotypes currently available have not been subjected to extensive selection and express high level of variability observed in the germplasm collection.[2,4,6,14-16] The genotypes mostly differ in their growth habits, morphological characteristics and chemical constituents and yield attributes (such as biomass production and seed yield) indicating that evolution has resulted in beneficial phenotypic variations in fenugreek that could be utilized for selective breeding purposes for further crop improvement.[2,14,15] However, one of the important limitations of the crop has been lack of variability in the existing populations for determinate growth habit. The number of available frost free days in western Canada is ~ 100 days and most fenugreek germplasm lines tested and found suitable for western Canadian growing conditions need ~120 days for producing high quantity and quality seeds due to their indeterminate growth habit. Hence, it was important for us to develop fast maturing fenugreek mutants with determinate growth habit and that can attain maturity within 100 days we opted for mutation breeding using ethyl methane sulfonate (EMS) at concentration dosages ranging from 10-300 mM and with incubation period varying between 2-24 hours.[17] We were successful in developing new breeding material for western Canada that exhibited early maturity duration and generated high quantity and quality of seed. Our work has been the first to report on successful application of mutation breeding in improving quantitative trait in this particular crop species.[17] We also investigated whether genotype X environment (G X E) interaction has any significant impact on the seed and forage yield when cultivated under short growing season of western Canada. We conducted two elaborate studies: first one involving 83 genotypes grown under both dryland and irrigated conditions of Lethbridge, Alberta for two years and a second study with five selected genotypes cultivated under seven separate environments scattered over the province of Alberta and British Columbia over five years, in western Canada. These studies indicated that improvement through phenotypic selection in forage and seed yield is possible but, would need selection using multiple locations and years due to strong G X E interaction. We concluded that significant improvement in fenugreek seed yield is achievable through selection for less variable seed size or for early maturity duration or determinate growth habits.[1,18] The doubling of somatic chromosome number often results in increase in plant vigour, the size of plant parts and seeds due to larger cell size, though it may decrease in seed production due to association with reduced frequency of viable gametes caused by irregularity of chromosome pairing.[19] With the hypothesis of getting vigorous and superior fenugreek plants for successful forage usage and plants with bigger seeds that may possess higher amount of oil and chemical constituents, we treated Tristar fenugreek seeds with colchicine, a natural alkaloid extracted from the autumn crocus, to double the chromosome number. Chromosome doubling was observed in some of the treated seeds; the tetraploid plants emerged from those seeds had larger leaves, longer pod length, vigorous growth and a greater height in comparison to untreated Tristar plants.[20] Any deleterious effect, such as poor seed setting which is a common phenomenon in induced polyploidy, was not found in successive generations of those tetraploid plants, which may be attributed to the inherent properties of the species fenugreek, and/or the appropriateness of the treatment doses and procedure that we used in that experiment.

A number of fenugreek diseases have been reported across the globe that is either abiotic or biotic in nature. The most common biotic agents infecting fenugreek are fungi, bacteria, viruses, insects and nematodes.[3,15] We also investigated potential fungal pathogens[21] and insect pets[22] of fenugreek under Canadian prairie agro-climatic conditions. The two major fungal diseases that affect fenugreek are powdery mildew caused by *Erysiphe polygoni* and Cercospora leaf spot caused by *Cercospora traversiana.*[15] We reported for the first time that powdery mildew caused by *Erysiphe polygoni* as one of the most serious fungal pathogens for reducing fenugreek yield in North America.[21] We are initiating an extensive and thorough study on the mood of action, extent to cause economic losses, prevention and control measures of *C. traversiana* on fenugreek putting more emphasis on screening tolerant ant resistant germplasms among the world accessions currently at Lethbridge Research Centre, Canada. Since, fenugreek is a relatively recent crop introduced in western Canada, it still does not have any serious insect pests at the present time. However, our study indicated that western flower thrips to be the most notorious under greenhouse conditions; while, *Lygus* bugs, and to a lesser extents alfalfa plant bugs and aphids to be detrimental to fenugreek yield under prairie field conditions.[22]

Medicinal, nutraceutical and functional food properties of fenugreek

The functional food values of fenugreek in conditioning health and nutrition in humans are well known. Fenugreek is extensively used as a spice in India and is known to possess a number of medicinal properties in alleviation of cardiovascular as well as hepatic disorders. Fenugreek has been reported as a medicinal plant in Indian Ayurveda and also in doctrines of ancient Chinese medicinal practices. Historical accounts indicate that fenugreek leaves and seeds were used for many medicinal purposes, such as treating mouth ulcers and chapped lips, cure of baldness, alleviation of abdominal and abscesses pain, treating arthritis, dropsy, heart disease, spleen and lever enlargement, kidney ailments among several others, in the subcontinent of India, Greece, Arab and China.[2,4] A wide range of medicinal properties has been attributed to fenugreek such as wound-healing, bust enhancement, enhanced lactation in weaning mothers (galactogogue), as an aphrodisiac, anti-diabetic, anti-hyperthyroidism, anti-cancer, gastro-protective, antioxidant, anti-pyretic, anti-nociceptive, anti-microbial, anti-helmintic, anti-sterility, anti-allergy, anti-inflammatory effects.[2] Medicinal and nutraceutical agents like steroidal sapogenins and mucilaginous fibres present in the seed and leaves of this legume plant contribute to anti-diabetic and hypocholesterolaemic properties attributed to the plant. Traditionally fenugreek leaves and seed have been used from time immemorial in preparing crude extracts and powders for different medicinal practices in different parts of the globe.[2]

In general, fenugreek contains three important phytochemicals with rich medicinal properties: 1) galactomannans, 2) sapogenins; and 3) 4-hydroxy isoleucine (Figure 2). Due to the presence of these chemicals fenugreek is currently rated higher among most commonly competing and well recognized nutraceuticals or health food products.[23,1] Galactomannan is a major polysaccharide molecule reported from fenugreek seeds contributing more than half of the seed weight and also forms an integral part of the cell wall.[4] The fenugreek galactomannan is unique due to the ~1:1 - 1.2:1 ratio of galactose to mannose (G:M) molecules.[3] This polysaccharide appears to be beneficial in controlling type 2 diabetes in animals as well as in humans.[24] In one human study, it has been found that taking 2.5 g of fenugreek per day for three months can significantly reduce cardiac risks. These benefits are linked to the presence of a group of water soluble fibres galactomannans having fat-seizing properties. The fibrous galactomannans directly bind to dietary fat and reduce its absorption into the body.

Fenugreek seed is an important source of steroidal sapogenins such as diosgenin, tigogenin, yamogenin, gitogenin, neotigogenin etc.[23,25] reported that steroidal sapogenins are extremely efficient in controlling hypocholesterolaemia. At present, natural diosgenin is procured and isolated from the tubers of certain wild Mexican yam (*Dioscorea*). But this process is both expensive and long, since these plants need many years to get to the marketable size of the tubers for economic extractions of diosgenin for use in pharmaceutical and neutraceutical formulations.[2] Fenugreek may turn into a feasible alternative for diosgenin yield because of its short growth cycle, cost-efficient production economy and fairly consistent yield attributes.[3,2] Fenugreek seeds possess furostanolic saponins which are believed to stimulate testosterone production by stimulating the brain to release gonadotropin-releasing hormone (GnRH) and luteinizing hormone (LH).

The amino acid isoleucine, a precursor of 4-hydroxyisoleucine has been reported for regulating insulin secretion, which shuttles nutrients as well as supplements directly into muscles, in the animal pancreas.[26] The presence of 4-hydroxyisoleucine in fenugreek seed is an added attribute for its ability to control the level of blood sugar, which helps decrease fat storage, in animal as well as human model studies.[2]

Fenugreek has antioxidant properties that can protect cells from damage, premature aging, ethanol toxicity and accumulation of damage resulting in cancer. The antioxidant properties of fenugreek seeds may have arose from their ability to regulate enzymes that control concentrations of oxidized products in cells.[27]

It is important to note that in recent time nutraceutical and functional food products have turned increasingly important commodities for health consumers globally and has aggressively transformed into a multi-billion dollar expanding industry. This huge surge of potential growth opens a big door for research and development in the nutraceutical and functional food arena. There is no doubt that fenugreek has pharmaceutical properties which can efficiently be utilized for medicinal and functional food purposes. Fenugreek with its exquisite medicinal and nutraceutical properties is a strong candidate for research in this area. In many advanced countries, fenugreek is now under active development for potential therapeutic products.[2,14,15,18,28] Present days, the medicinal components extracted from leaves and seeds of fenugreek are being introduced as nutraceuticals and functional foods in chewing gums, candies, baked goods, ice creams, teas, soft drinks and other food supplements. In very recent times, the nutraceutical and medicinal value of fenugreek has become important in pharmaceuticals and functional food industries in Canada. There is growing recognition of the potential role for nutraceuticals and dietary supplements to reduce health risks and improve health quality. In the global marketplace nutraceuticals and functional foods have become a multi-billion dollar industry and estimates within Canada suggest that the Canadian nutraceutical and functional food industries have potential to grow to 50 billion US dollar.[28] Specialty crops like fenugreek are drawing attention of producers to meet the demands for functional food additives and natural health products in Canada.[28]

For proper commercialization of *T. foenum-graecum* L. as an effective nutraceutical and pharmaceutical important crop, the most critical problem is the lack of adapted cultivars to different agro-climates over the world. Therefore, now it is the main role and challenge for plant breeders to develop fenugreek cultivars with improved quality and productivity characteristics adapted to the agro-climatic zones. Appropriate management and developmental researches may turn this 'old world crop' as an important source of healthful foods and food supplements for the people of the 'new world'. We see an enormous opportunity to work towards developing fenugreek cultivars rich in different nutraceutical and functional products locally adapted to specific environment and locality. The plant has already shown quite impressive growth in the nutraceutical and functional food markets of USA and has the potentiality to grow into a much bigger consumer product in there long run.[28] We believe that by exploiting eco-genetic variations within natural population of fenugreek for nutraceutical and functional food potentialities we would be able to help in generating the niche markets distinctive to Canada and North America as well as generate needs for the international markets in Japan, USA and European Union. Being not genetically modified, this crop has enormous potentiality for its marketability in the western hemisphere as forage, nutraceutical and functional food in the not so distant future. With respect to food safety and food quality issues fenugreek, no doubt has a bigger advantage over other competing crops in seizing the new health food industry and market.

Fenugreek is reported as a gifted herb in many literatures as it possess insecticidal, nematicidal, molluscicidal and antimicrobial properties.[2] Fenugreek itself is an insect tolerant crop; moreover, it provides effective control against stored grain insect pests. Dried fenugreek leaves are used in India to repel harmful insect pests from stored grain. Fenugreek seed and leaf extract mixed with stored grain have been reported to kill pest like *Tribolium castaneum* (Herbst) and *Acanthoscelides obtectus* (Say), and can successfully kill the larvae of phytopathogenic nematode *Meloidogyne javanica.*[2]

Anti-microbial properties

Fenugreek seed and leaf extracts were reported to have widespread anti-microbial activity against both gram positive and gram negative bacteria,[29] although other researchers have reported that extracts of fenugreek seeds collected from India were failure to prevent growth of either bacteria or yeast. Since, high levels of antimicrobial compounds within the leaves and stems of forage crops could result in negative weight gain in livestock and minimize returns to livestock industry by killing ruminant bacteria and yeast, we conducted an experiment to examine the effect of aqueous and ethanol extracts from the leaves and seeds of 75 fenugreek world accessions on the growth of some enteric bacteria and yeast which are commonly found within digestive tracts of most animals. None of the accessions we used in our study possessed any anti-microbial activity against those bacteria and yeast suggesting the superior efficacy of fenugreek forage cultivars to maximize returns to livestock industries supporting weight gain in livestock.[29]

Anti-neoplastic properties

Leukemia represents a heterogeneous group of neoplasm arising from malignant transformation of haematopoietic cells i.e. blood forming cells. It is a disease of blood forming tissues in which the bone marrow is always involved and is characterized by overabundance of one cell type, usually an immature leukocyte.

Leukemia is the most common childhood malignancy, representing 30% of all childhood cancers in children under the age of 15 years.[30] B type Chronic Lymphocytic Leukemia (B-CLL) is the most common leukemia in the western world. These leukemic cells are apparently derived form the CD5 expressing B cell subset. B-CLL remains an incurable illness and there is no survival benefit to early intervention.[31] So there is an urgency to cure this incurable leukemia. Many anticancer therapies currently in use are inadequate not only in terms of their therapeutic efficacy but also because they have undesirable side effects. On the other hand, certain dietary constituents known as phytochemicals have been shown to exhibit growth-suppressive activity and chemo-preventive properties against various types of cancers[32] without the adverse side effects normally associated with current chemotherapies. Fenugreek plant extract comprises precious compounds which have shown cardiotonic, anticholeserolaemic, hypoglycaemic, diuretic, antichloristic, and hypertensive activity. As a medicinal plant, fenugreek has also been studied and employed in the treatment of cancer for its potential effectiveness as a cancer chemo-preventive by cancer researchers. It is thought that fenugreek may help to prevent cancer by raising the levels of vitamin C, vitamin E, and other antioxidants in the bloodstream. One of its constituents is an alkaloid called trigonelline [2] which has shown potential for use in cancer and neoplasm therapy. Fenugreek may be a promising protective medicinal herb for consideration in complementary therapy in cancer patients under chemotherapeutic interventions.[33] The anti-leukemic effect of *T. foenum-graecum* seed extract has been evaluated in few B-CLL patients, where two strains showed a robust induction of apoptosis. This study will have a major impact in the identification of new drugs in curing the incurable CLL. Fenugreek galactomannans were found significantly effective for activation of phagocytosis in rat peritoneal macrophages, proliferation and IgM secretion in human–human hybridoma, HB4C5 cells which are the human–human hybridomas producing monoclonal antibodies against human lung cancer.[34] The fenugreek constituent diosgenin is reported to have potential as a novel colon cancer preventive agent. The preventive efficacy of dietary fenugreek seed and its major steroidal saponin constituent, diosgenin, were evaluated on azoxymethane-induced rat colon carcinogenesis during initiation and promotion stages. Study results indicated that diosgenin inhibits tumour cell growth and induces apoptosis in the HT-29 human colon cancer cell by inhibition of bcl-2 and by induction of caspase-3 protein expression line in a dose-dependent manner.[35]

Antioxidant properties

Over the past three decades there has been an almost overwhelming increase in the volume of scientific and medical literature relating nutritional factors to most of mankind's degenerative and killer diseases. Paralleling this growth is the evidence that oxidation generated free radical reactions are involved in most, if not at all, of these disorders. Free radicals are highly reactive unpaired electrons which cause oxidation of metabolites in the body resulting in cell death and tissue injury.[36] Oxidative damage at the cellular or sub-cellular level is now considered to be a major event in disease processes like coronary vascular disease, inflammatory disease, diabetes, carcinogenesis and aging. Reactive oxygen radicals are detrimental to cells at both membrane and genetic levels.[37]

Free radicals arc formed as a part of body's normal metabolic process. Synthetic (xenobiotic) chemicals, radiation, X-rays, pollution and even stress can produce these damaging entities. The chemicals known to produce free radicals include chlorinated hydrocarbons, aromatic hydrocarbons, industrial acids, solvents, most pesticides and herbicides, preservatives in foods, printing pigments and inks and other industrial chemicals, fragrances and perfume vehicles, cosmetic vehicles and cosmetics, pollutants in air and water, many if not all pharmacological agents used in medicine and anaesthetics, etc. Even the transitional metal catalysts iron and copper, which are ubiquitous, have a most powerful generating effect on chain initiating radicals. Chemical mobilization of fat stores under various conditions such as lactation, exercise, fever, infection and even fasting, can result in increased radical activity and damage in particular to the immune and nervous systems.[36]

Seed administration of **fenugreek** reduced the increase in the levels of biomarkers of oxidative stress in the liver of rats dosed with EtOH.[38] Later on the same group also showed that treatment of cells with EtOH led to significantly higher release of thiobarbituric acid-reactive substances (TBARS) as compared with untreated control cells. Ethanolic extract of fenugreek powder caused a dose-dependent reduction of TBARS production.[39]

Dietary fenugreek seed has been shown to counter the increased lipid peroxidation and alterations in the content of circulating antioxidant molecules, such as glutathione, β-carotene, α-tocopherol and scavenge reactive oxygen species.[27] A methanolic extract of fenugreek seeds exhibited scavenging of hydroxyl radicals, inhibition of hydrogen peroxide-induced lipid peroxidation in rat liver mitochondria, 2,22 -Diphenyl-1-picrylhydrazyl (DPPH) and 2,22 -azinobis-(3-ethylbenzothiazoline-6-sulfonic acid) (ABTS) radical scavenging activity.[40]

Oxidative stress may be a common route linking the diverse complications of diabetes with the mechanism of its pathogenesis. Some of the mechanisms that lead to oxidative stress, in addition to enzymatic and oxidative glycation of proteins, are metabolic stresses arising from alterations in energy metabolism of cells, changes in the polyol pathway, the changes in antioxidant enzyme levels, cellular damages due to radiation and some inflammatory reactions.[41] Peroxidative tissue damage has been observed in the pathogenesis and complications of both Type I and Type II diabetes. Increased oxidative damage has been obtained in the kidneys and hearts of diabetic rats during diabetes.[42]

With the premise that oxygen free radicals may be responsible for the severity and complications of diabetes, the level of antioxidant enzymes catalase (CAT), superoxide dismutase (SOD) and glutathione peroxidase (GPx) as well as the oxidative damage were examined[43] in the tissues of control, diabetic and treated rats. After 3 weeks of diabetes, the activity of CAT was significantly increased in heart in diabetes (about 6-fold) but decreased in liver. The SOD activity decreased significantly in liver but increased in brain. The activity of GPx decreased significantly in liver and increased in kidney. A significant increase was reported in oxidative damage in heart and kidney and a small increase in brain with decrease in liver and muscle. Fenugreek administration to diabetic animals showed a reversal of the disturbed antioxidant levels and peroxidative damage.[43]

The protective effect of the aqueous extract of the seeds on the activity of calcium-dependent adenosinetriphosphatase (Ca^{2+}-ATPase) in liver homogenate in the presence of Fe^{2+}/ascorbate *in vitro* was also investigated. Ca^{2+}-ATPase activity in liver was protected by the aqueous extract to nearly 80%. The findings suggest that the soluble portion of the seeds could be responsible for the antioxidant property.

The antioxidant effect of fenugreek leaves was evaluated in the streptozotocin-induced diabetic rat model.[44] The antioxidant effect was evaluated by estimating TBARS and reduced glutathione, and measuring the activities of catalase and superoxide dismutase in liver, heart and kidney in diabetic rats. Fenugreek leaf powder supplementation significantly lowered lipid peroxidation and increased the antioxidant system in diabetic rats. The effect at a dose of 1 g/kg of body weight of fenugreek leaf powder was similar to that of glibenclamide. From the published works it is quite clear that fenugreek shows an encouraging antioxidant property that can be exploited for treatment/reversal of complications of diabetes and other ailments.

Fenugreek and clinical trials

Most of the investigations on medicinal values of fenugreek have been undertaken in rats.[45] Fenugreek seeds have been shown to have medicinal values of treating alcohol induced hepatic disorders in humans and also have hypoglycemic and hypocholesterolaemic effects on type 1 and type 2 diabetes mellitus patients and experimental diabetic animals.[46] In an *in vitro* study to determine if galactomannan affects intestinal glucose uptake in genetically determined lean and obese rats, it was reported that galactomannan, a soluble fiber can reduce postprandial blood glucose response.[23]

However, either community based nutrition and health surveys or the clinical trials through case and control method in human patients suffering from diabetes and hypertension or any hepatic functional disorders and the assessment of medicinal values of fenugreek are very less. Sharma et al.[47] examined the effect of fenugreek seeds on blood glucose and the serum lipid profile was evaluated in insulin-dependent (Type I) diabetic patients. Their results showed that the fenugreek diet significantly reduced fasting blood sugar and improved the glucose tolerance test. The effects of fenugreek seeds on glycemic control and insulin resistance in mild to moderate type 2 diabetes mellitus were also evaluated by a double blind placebo controlled study.[48] These studies reported that the adjunct use of fenugreek seeds improves glycemic control and decreases insulin resistance in mild to moderate type-2 diabetic patients. In a similar study[49] conducted in larger sample size and continued for a much longer period in randomized human patients of type 2 diabetes, the medicinal values of fenugreek to reduce and to control the blood sugar level have been established. There is also a favorable effect on hypertriglyceridemia. In patients with non-insulin dependent diabetes mellitus and associated chronic liver disease, plasma levels of glucose, insulin and triglycerides are high, lipid peroxidation is increased and natural antioxidant reserves are reduced. Lirussi et al.[50] reported that oral administration of silybin-β-cyclodextrin in such patients causes a significant decrease in both glucose and triglyceride plasma levels. A recent study presents evidence that the major isomer of 4-hydroxyisoleucine, an atypical branched-chain amino acid derived from fenugreek, is responsible for the effects of this plant on glucose and lipid metabolism.[51]

Conclusions

One of the most common observations from the published literature in the area related to value of fenugreek for nutrition and levels of phytochemicals etc has been that the results are inconsistent. This is however not unique to fenugreek studies. Results from studies conducted on plant products in different research institutions are conflicting and so do not get the attention they deserve. These results are some times so inconsistent that people have difficulty believing the conclusions drawn from them. We have observed that the same genotype of fenugreek produces different levels of a chemical(s) when grown under different environments. This strong G X E effect is consistent in several crop species and fenugreek is not an exception to this particular pattern. Research results from our laboratory indicate that there is strong G X E effect for the phytochemicals anti-microbial properties[16,29]. Fenugreek genotypes also exhibit G X E interaction for other traits such as biomass production, seed yield, maturity duration and disease resistance. It is therefore important that attempts be made to develop adapted cultivars with stable phytochemical levels so that the crop can be utilized to its potential. A multidisciplinary research group is currently working in India and Canada to identify important genotypes with essential nutraceutical and medicinal properties so that the crop can be used to its potential.

References

1. S.K. Basu, S.N. Acharya and J.E. Thomas, Production of high quality fenugreek (*Trigonella foenum-graecum* L.). (MSc Thesis), (VDM Verlag, Germany, (2009).

2. S.N. Acharya, J.E. Thomas and S.K. Basu, *Crop Sci.* **48**, 841-853, (2008).

3. G..A. Petropoulos, Fenugreek –The genus *Trigonella*, 1st ed. (Taylor and Francis, London and New York, (2002), pp. 1-127.

4. S.N. Acharya, J.E. Thomas and S.K. Basu, Fenugreek: An annual forage legume and its role in preservation of water quality and conservation of water. In Proc. Ann. Workshop for the Oldman River Basin Water Quality Initiative, 7th, 2 Mar. 2004. Lethbridge, AB, Canada , (2004).

5. V. Kumar, The secret benefits of spices and condiments, (New dawn press, New Delhi, India, pp. 58-59, (2006).

6. S. Acharya, A. Srichamoren, S. Basu, B. Ooraikul and T. Basu, Improvement in the nutraceutical properties of fenugreek (*Trigonella foenum-graecum* L.) p. 45, In Proc. World Congress on Clinical Nutrition, 10th, 30 Nov.–3 Dec. 2004. Phuket, Thailand , (2004).

7. C.D. Darlington and A.P. Wylie, Chromosome Atlas of Flowering Plants. 1st ed. George Allen and Unwin Ltd., London, , p.161, (1945).

8. F. Rosengarten, The Book of Spices ,Livingstone, Wynnewood, Pennsylvania, USA, (1969).

9. G..L. Yadav and P.D. Kumawat, Haryana *J. Hort. Sci.* **32**, 147-148, (2003).

10. M.H. Abd-Ala and S.A. Omar, *Biol. Fertil. Soil.* **26**, 58-65, (1998).

11. S.K. Basu, S.N. Acharya and J.E. Thomas, KMITL *Sci. & Tech. J.* **8**, 1-7, (2008).

12. B. Dey and R.C. Srivastava, *Biol. Memiors.* **30**, 78-85, (2004).

13. S.K. Basu, S.N. Acharya and J.E. Thomas, *Proc. Multi. Grad. Res. Conf.* **1**, 44-50 ,(2007).

14. S.N. Acharya, J.E. Thomas and S.K. Basu, *Biodiversity*. **7**, 27-30, (2006).

15. S.N. Acharya, J. E. Thomas, R. Prasad and S.K. Basu, Diseases of fenugreek (*Trigonella foenum-graecum* L.) and control measures with special emphasis on fungal diseases. In: Arya, A. P. and Perelló, A. E. (eds.) Management of fungal pathogens: Current trends and progress (CABI, Nosworthy Way, Wallingford, Oxon, UK, 2009). (in press).

16. W.G. Taylor, H.L. Zulyniak, K.W. Richards, S.N. Acharya, S. Bittman and J.L. Elder, *J. Agric. Food Chem.* **50**, 5994-5997, (2002).

17. S.K. Basu, S.N. Acharya and J.E. Thomas, *Euphytica* 160, 249-258, (2008).

18. S.K. Basu, S.N. Acharya, D. Friebel, M. Bandara and J.E. Thomas, *Aust. J. Agri. Res.*, (2009). (currently under revision).

19. W.R. Fehr, Principles of cultivar development (Macmillan publishing company, New York, 1987) Vol. I, pp. 59-62.

20. S.K. Basu, S.N. Acharya and J.E. Thomas, Proc. Multi. Grad. Res. Conf. **1**, 37-43 ,(2007).

21. S.K. Basu, S.N. Acharya and J.E. Thomas, *J. Mycopathol. Res.* **44**, 253-256, (2006).

22. S.K. Basu, S.N. Acharya, H.A. Cárcamo and J.E. Thomas, *J. Environ. & Sociobiol.* 3, 1-7, (2006).

23. A. Srichamroen, A.B. Thomson, C.J. Field and T.K. Basu, *Nutr. Res.* **29**, 49-54, (2009).

24. V. Vats, S.P. Yadav and J.K. Grover, *J. Ethanopharmocol.* **28**, 1-6 , (2003).

25. M.A. McAnuff, F.O. Omoruyi, E.Y.S.A. Morrison and H.N. *Nutr. Res.* **22**, 1427-1434, (2002).

26. C. Broca, M. Manteghetti, R. Gross, Y. Baissac, M. Jacob, P. Petit, P., Y. Sauvaire, and G. Ribes, *Eur. J. Pharmacol.* **390**, 339-345, (2000).

27. S. N. Acharya and J. E. Thomas, Advances in medicinal plant research. (Research Signpost, Kerala, India, 2007) pp. 81-122.

28. S.K. Basu, J.E. Thomas and S.N. Acharya, *Aust. J. Basic Appl. Sci.* **1**, 637-649, (2007).

29. J.E. Thomas, S.K. Basu and S.N. Acharya, *Can. J. Plant Sci.* **86**, 727-732, (2006).

30. S. Pal, S. Ghosh, S. Bandyopadhyay, C.N. Mandal, S. Bandhyopadhyay, D.K. Bhattacharya and C. Mandal, *Inter. J. Cancer.* **11**, 270-277 , (2004).

31. E. Montserrat and C. Rozman, *Annals. Oncol.* **6**, 219, (1995).

32. Y.J. Surh, *Nat. Rev. Cancer.* **3**, 768–80 ,(2003).

33. K. Bhatia, M. Kaur, F. Atif, M. Ali, H. Rehman, S. Rahman and S. Raisuddin, *Food Chem. Toxicol.* **44**, 1744-50, (2006).

34. H.P. Ramesh, K. Yamaki and T. Tsushida, *Carbohydr. Polym.* **50**, 79-831 , (2002).

35. J. Raju, J.M.R. Patlolla, M.V. Swamy and C.V. Rao, *Biomarkers Prev.* **13**, 1392-1398 , (2004).

36. K.H. Cheeseman and T.F. *British Medical Bulletin*, **49**, 481-493, (1993).

37. K. Srinivasan, *Food Rev. Int.* **22**, 203-224, (2006).

38. V. Thirunavukkarasu, C.V. Anuradha and P. Viswanathan, *Phytother. Res.* **17**, 737-743, (2003).

39. S. Kaviarasan, K. Vijayalakshmi and C.V. Anuradha, *Plant Foods Hum. Nutr.* **59**, 143-7, (2004).

40. S. Kaviarasan, G.H. Naik, R. Gangabhagirathi, C.V. Anuradha and K.I. Priyadarsini, *Food Chem.* **103**, 31-37, (2007).

41. S. Genet, R.K. Kale and N.Z. Baquer, *Ind. J. Exp. Biol.* **37**, 200-202, (1999).

42. P.S.M. Prince, V.P. Menon and L. Pari, *J. Ethnopharmacol.* **61**, 1-7, (1998).

43. S. Genet, R.K. Kale and N.Z. Baquer, *Mol. Cell. Biochem.* **236**, 7-12, (2002).

44. B. Annida and P.S.M. Prince, *J. Medic. Food.* **8**, 382-385, (2005).

45. W.L. Xue, X.S. Li, J. Zhang, Y.H. Liu, Z.L. Wang and R.J. Zhang, *Asia Pac. J. Clin. Nutr.* **16**, 422-426, (2007).

46. S. Kaviarasan and C.V. Anuradha, *Pharmazie.* **62**, 299-304, (2007).

47. R.D. Sharma, T.C. Raghuram, N.S. Rao, *Eur. J. Clin. Nutr.* **44**, 301-306, (1990).

48. A. Gupta, R. Gupta and B. Lal, *J. Assoc. Physicians India*. **49,** 1057-1061, (2001).

49. V.L. Roberts, J. Stewart, M. Issa, B. Lake and R. Melis, *Clin. Ther*. **27**, 1535-1547, (20050.

50. F. Lirussi, A. Beccarello, G. Zanette, A. De Monte, V. Donadon, M. Velussi and G. Crepaldi, *Diabetes Nutr. Metab*. **15,** 222-231, (2002).

51. L. Jetté, L. Harvey, K. Eugeni and N. Levens, *Curr. Opin. Investig. Drugs*. **10**, 353-358, (2009).

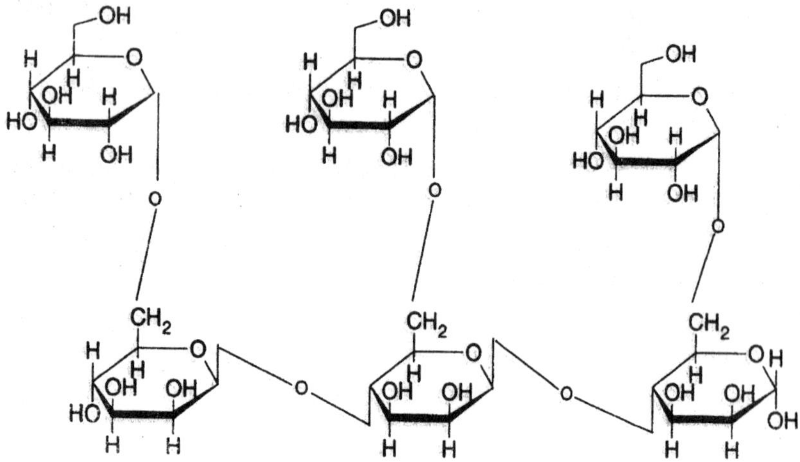

1. Galactomannan

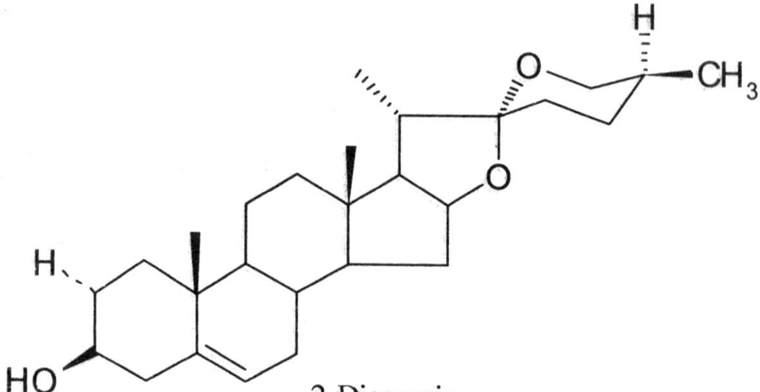

2. Diosgenin

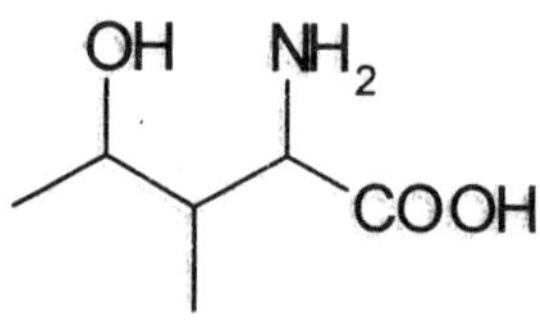

3. 4-Hydroxyisoleucine

Figure 2. Chemical structures of important phytochemicals reported from fenugreek.

Exploring the CNS Active Potentials of Some Indian Spices

N. Satheesh Kumar, Pulok K. Mukherjee, S. Bhadra, S. Pommusankar

Conventional medicine is now pursuing the use of natural products including herbs to provide the support that the disorders needs on a daily basis. Many of these herbs have been evaluated in clinical studies and are currently being investigated phytoconstituents to understand their actions. An attempt has been made through this article to review the CNS active potentials of some Indian Spices which are pharmacologically established as the source of potential for new drugs. In this review, the ethno botanical information on Spices specifically on CNS related disorders like epilepsy, depression, age-related dementia etc were discussed in recent scientific studies conducted on some of these spices are reviewed for CNS disorders. This will help to explore and initiate research on isolation of bioactive compounds from natural resources to treat CNS disorders.

Introduction

Spices are usually a dried seed, fruit, root, bark or vegetative substance used in nutritionally insignificant quantities as a food additive for the purpose of flavoring. Spices are defined as a strongly flavored or aromatic substance of vegetable origin, obtained from tropical plants, commonly used as a condiment.

Spices have been extensively used in history for flavouring and seasoning foods, beverages and medicines.[1-4] The spicy history started with the adventures of Vasco da-gama about 5000 years ago. In ancient times, spices were as precious as gold; and as significant as medicines, preservatives and perfumes. India played a significant role in the global trade of spices. India produces around 2.75 million tones of different spices valued at approximately 4.2 billion US $, and holds the premier position in the world spices market. Plants used as spices and condiments are usually aromatic and pungent.[5] Iwu[6] (1993) had reported that these plants owe these properties to the presence of varying types of essential oils. It is also credited with many health benefits like aiding digestion, a disinfectant, and rich in fiber, minerals and vitamins. Several pharmacological studies on spices like antioxidant, anti-inflammatory, anti-amyloid, hypocholeterolaemic, anti neurodegenerative etc. activities have also been reported. There are quite a few leads available for the treatment of neurodegenerative diseases and but the clinical outcome of these agents are not always convincing.[7,8] This is the prime driving force behind the investigation of natural sources for the best safest remedy. And the spices came into the focus, as some reports revealed that consumptions of spices keep a man away from several Central Nervous System (CNS) disorders, namely Alzheimer's. This information is further intended to contribute in the documentation and provision of accurate record of indigenous knowledge, use and conservation of these plants, and their subsequent integration in the efforts towards the development of natural product and indigenous health care management, Especially for the CNS ailments.[9,10] The present review highlights some of the important spices in Indian System of medicine, which have potential CNS activities.

2. Some Indian spices and their activity on CNS

Spices are not only known to add taste, aroma and flavor to the food, but also for their medicinal properties. The spices have been used since centuries in traditional medicinal systems like

Ayurveda, Traditional Chinese Medicine (TCM), Unani medicine etc. the medicinal values of spices have been documented in many ancient literatures. Sometimes they are used in formulation with other ingredients as principle ingredient or alone. Till today the some homemade remedies includes spices. As the Phytochemical techniques progressed and the newer technologies invaded, facilitated the thorough evaluation of phytoconstituents of the spices. It revealed so many important classes of natural chemical entities present in the plant. These constituents have great potential to treat CNS disorders. The available treatments for CNS disorders with the synthetic drugs bring about life threatening side effects. To overcome this serious problem researchers in the phytomedicine field are always in search of potential lead molecules from natural sources. Here we discussed some of the spices evaluated scientifically and reported for their CNS related activities.

Artemisia dracunculus L.

The essential oil obtained from the aerial parts of the plant was studied for anticonvulsant potential. The essential oil showed antiseizure activity in both maximal electroshock and pentylenetetrazole model.[11] Stafford et al 2005[12] reported some plants traditionally used in South Africa as sedatives or CNS-related ailments (Table 1).

Capsicum annum **L.**

Capsicum annum belongs to family Solanaceae. Loizzo et al 2008[13] tested the in vitro hypoglycemic and anti-acetylcholinesterase activities of hot pepper fruits, it showed (IC_{50}) = 84.30 microg/mL) inhibition. Szabó et al 2004[14] investigated a new immunotherapeutic approaches to induce functionally beneficial anti-Aβ antibody responses in different transgenic animal models of AD (Table 1).

Coriandrum sativum **L.**

The anxiolytic effect of aqueous extract of *Coriandrum sativum* L. (10, 25, 50, 100 mg/kg, i.p.) was studied in animal model. The aqueous extract at 100 mg/kg showed an anxiolytic effect[15] (Table 1).

Curcuma Longa L.

A phenolic compound curcumin a yellow pigment in curry spice isolated from the roots have shown anti-inflammatory, antioxidant, anticarcinogenic, antiviral, and anti infectious activities associated with Alzheimer's disease. Ahmed and Gilani 2009[16] evaluate acetylcholinesterase (AChE) inhibitory and memory enhancing activities with Curcuminoids (a mixture of curcumin, bisdemethoxycurcumin and demethoxycurcumin). IC50 value of bisdemethoxycurcumin, demethoxycurcumin and curcumin is 19.67, 16.84, 33.14 67.69 μM respectively. Curcumin has also potent anti-amyloidogenic effects on beta-amyloid for Alzheimer's disease.[17] Kumar et al 2007[18] studied cognitive impairment and oxidative stress in rats against colchicines. Further behaviours and serotonergic receptor-coupled AC-cAMP signal pathway in rats were investigated[19] (Table 1).

Elettaria cardamom L.

A novel ayurvedic formulation 'Unmadnashak Ghrita' (UG) containing *Elettaria cardamom*, *Ferula narthex*, *Gardenia gummifera*, *Bacopa monneri*, and cow's ghee (clarified butter fat) were developed for their neuropharmacological activities. UG formulation showed CNS depressant activity and anticonvulsant activity in mice.[20] Joshi and Parle[21] studied the nootropic effects of Brahmi rasayana (BR) a memory enhancer (Table 1).

Murraya koenigii L.

Murraya koenigii commonly known as curry patta belongs to the family Rutaceae. The leaves of *Murraya koenigii* are also used as antidiabetic, antioxidant, antimicrobial, anti-inflammatory, hepatoprotective, anti-hypercholesterolemic, Nootropic and

Antiamnesic activities. The cognitive functions of *Murraya koenigii* leaves were investigated on total serum cholesterol level and brain cholinesterase activity in young and aged mice. The memory scores were measured using various exteroceptive and interoceptive behavioral models and it showed significant dose-dependent improvement in the memory.[22] Further the nootropic effect were studied form *Murraya koenigii* leaves in young and aged rats[23] (Table 1).

Trigonella foenum graecum L.

Trigonella foenum graecum belongs to the family Fabaceae. It has been used since ancient times in Indian folklore medicine for its many medicinal properties. TFG is reported to possess anxiolytic, nootropic, immunomodulatory and hypoglycemic properties. Different extract of *Trigonella foenum graecum*, fenugreek oil, diosgenin and trigonelline were tested for neuropharmacological activity. All the extracts, diosgenin and trigonelline showed significant central nervous system stimulant activity.[24]The antidepressant effect of methanolic extract of fenugreek seeds was studied and it significantly reduced the immobility during FST and TST in a dose dependant manner.[25] Further Mohan et al 2006[26] studied nootropic and anxiolytic activity of fenugreek seeds (Table 1).

Tamarindus indica L.

Moshi et al 2005[27] reported some plants traditionally used in Tanzania to treat epilepsy. *Tamarindus indica* L. (Leguminosae) roots were boil with water, one cup of the decoction were taken daily to treat epilepsy (Table 1).

Zingiber officinale L.

Zingiber officinale Roscoe is commonly known as ginger and used as a 'rasayana' drug in the traditional system of medicine for centuries to treat dementia in South Asia.

The rhizomes and stems of ginger have assumed significant roles in Chinese, Japanese, and Indian medicine since the 1500s. Ginger root is widely used around the world as a spice or food additive. The ginger extract significantly improved learning and memory in young mice and also reversed the amnesia induced by diazepam and scopolamine, it also reversed aging induced amnesia due to natural aging of mice[28] (Table 1).

Secondary metabolites responsible for CNS activities

Plant secondary metabolites are a generic term used for more than 30,000 different substances which are exclusively produced by plants. There is considerable interest in the screening of plant and other natural product extracts in modern drug discovery programs, since structurally novel chemotypes with potent and selective biological activity may be obtained.[29,30] A consideration of biological activity in addition to the isolation and structure elucidation stages in a phytochemical investigation may add a great deal to the overall scientific significance of the work. Phytochemists may gain considerable information by using panels of simple bioassays and/or more specialized in vitro bioassays to follow each step of a purification procedure.[31-33] In recent years there has been an upsurge in interest from other disciplines, related to the realisation that secondary metabolites are dietary components that may have a considerable impact on human health, and to the development of gene technology that permits modulation of the contents of desirable and undesirable components. Curcumin (**1**) a poly phenol isolated from *Curcuma Longa* L. for acetylcholinesterase inhibitory activity.[16] Diosgenin (**2**) and trigonelline (**3**) showed significant central nervous system stimulant activity.[24] The essential oil extracted from *Artemisia dracunculus* namely camphene (**4**), linalool (**5**), α-pinene (**6**), β-pinene (**7**), eugenol (**8**), limonene (**9**), camphor (**10**), borneol (**11**) and estragole (**12**) tested for their acetylcholinesterase (AChE) inhibitory activity.[34]

Scope of novel lead finding from spices

Spices are one of the most extensively used in India for its aroma and several other medicinal properties. In recent years, there has been an emphasis on secondary metabolites in relation to dietary components, which may have a considerable impact on human health. The majority of the spices constitute important bioactive secondary metabolites which possess versatile pharmacological and medicinal properties. In spite of the various challenges encountered in the medicinal plant based drug discovery, natural products isolated from plants will still remain an essential component in the search for new medicines. Ayurvedic practitioners and researchers in medical sciences can help to improve this medicine by increasing their involvement and contribution. The diverse genetic resources and associated rich traditional knowledge available in India form the strong basis for bioprospecting. Proper utilization of these resources and tools in bioprospecting will certainly help in discovering novel lead molecules from plants by employing modern drug discovery techniques and the coordinated efforts of various disciplines. Several authors are currently being undertaken to isolate the active compounds by bioassay-guided fractionation from the spices that showed CNS related activity during screening. Therefore, these scientific investigations may be utilized to develop drugs for these CNS disorders. Further research is deserved to isolate the compounds responsible for the observed biological activity.

Conclusion

The medicinal values of the spices are as gorgeous as the history of spice. Since the adventure of vendors from different parts of the world attracted toward the India for spices through the spice route, the journey and the mystery about its aptitude also started. The people used to be powerful with the ownership of pepper. Still today the mystery of the spices has not been totally uncovered. Many important therapeutic have already been discussed and many are still to be revealed. It needs a great passion go work in this area of spices and explore magical dimensions. Moreover, spices can serve as storage of novel leads for CNS ailments, and waiting for exploration.

References

1. J.W. Parry, Spices-Morphology, Histology, Chemistry Vol. II Food Trade Press Ltd London. (1969).
2. J.D. Dziezak, Innovative food trends: Species. *Food Technology* **43(1)**: 102 – 116, (1989).
3. N.P. Manandhar, *J. of Herbs, Spices and Medicinal Plants* **3**: 71-77. (1995).
4. P.K. Mukherjee, Quality Control on Herbal Drugs. Business Horizons Limited:New Delhi 2002, pp. 1–37 (2002).
5. S.C. Achinewu, Aniena, M.I. and Obomanu, F.G., *J. African Med. Plants*, ,**18**:135-139, (1995).
6. M.M. Iwu, Handbook of African Medicinal Plants, Boca Raton CKC Press, 435 pp. (1993).
7. P K. Mukherjee, *Drug Inf J* **35**:623-631. (2001).
8. P K Mukherjee, K Maiti, K Mukherjee, PJ Houghton. *J Ethnopharmacol*, **106**:1-28. (2006).
9. P.K. Mukherjee, V. Kumar, N.S. Kumar, M. Heinrich, *J Ethnopharmacol*, **120(3)**, 291-301, (2008).
10. P.K. Mukherjee, V. Kumar, M. Mal, P.J. **Houghton,** *Phytomedicine*, **14(4)**:289-300. (2007).
11. M. Sayyah, L. Nadjafnia, M. Kamalinejad, *J Ethnopharmacol*, **94(2-3)**:283-7. (2004).
12. G.I. Stafford, A.K. Jäger, J. van Staden, *J Ethnopharmacol*, **100(1-2)**:210-5. (2005).
13. M.R. Loizzo, R. Tundis, F. Menichini, G.A. Statti, F. Menichini, *J Med Food.*,**11(1):**184-9. (2008).
14. B. Szabó, K. Hori, A. Nakajima, N. Sasagawa, Y. Watanabe, S. Ishiura, *Assay and Drug Development Technologies,* **2 (4),** 383-388. (2004).
15. M. Emamghoreishi, M. Khasaki, M.F. Aazam, *J Ethnopharmacol*, **96 (3) :** 365-70. (2005).

16. T. Ahmed, A.H. Gilani, *Pharmacol. Biochem. Behav.*, **91(4):**554-559. (2009).

17. J. M. Ringman, S.A. Frautschy, G.M. Cole, D.L. Masterman, J.L. Cummings, *Current Alzheimer Research,* **2 (2)**, 131-136, (2005).

18. A. Kumar, P.S. Naidu, N. Seghal, S.S. Padi, *J Med Food.* **10(3):**486-94, (2007).

19. Y. C. Li, F.M. Wang, Y. Pan, L.Q. Qiang, G. Cheng, W.Y. Zhang, L.D. Kong. *Biol. Psychiatry,* **33(3),** 435-449. (2009).

20. G. S. Achliya, S.G. Wadodkar, A.K. Dorle; *J. Ethnopharmacol.*, **94(1)**:77-83. (2004).

21. H. Joshi, M.Parle, *Evid Based Complement Alternat Med.*, **3(1):**79-85. (2006)a.

22. M. Vasudevan, M. Parle, *Phytother Res.*; **23(3):**308-16, (2009).

23. M. Vasudevan, M. Parle, S. Sengottuvelu, T. Shanmugapriya, *Nootropic International journal oriental pharmacy and experimental medicine.* **8(4),**365-373. (2008).

24. B. Natarajan, A. Muralidharan, R. Satish, Dhananjayan, *Journal of Natural Remedies,* **7 (1),**160-165, (2007).

25. V. S. Pawar, S. Hugar, B. Gawade, R.N. Patil, *Pharmacologyonline,* **1**: 455-465, (2008).

26. M. Mohan, A. Banekar, T. Birdi, P. Bharambe, S. Kaul, A. Patel, *Journal of Natural Remedies,* ,**6(2)**, 153—156. (2006).

27. M.J. Moshi, G.A. Kagashe, Z.H. Mbwambo, *J Ethnopharmacol.*, **97(2):**327-336, (2005).

28. H. Joshi, M. Parle, *Zingiber Officinale*: *Afr. J. Trad. CAM.*, **3 (1):** 64 – 74, (2006)b.

29. P. K. Mukherjee, A. Wahile, *J Ethnopharmacol.*;**103**:25-35. (2006).

30. S. Rai, A. Wahile, K. Mukherjee, B.P. Saha, P.K. Mukherjee, *J Ethnopharmacol*; **104**, 322-327. (2006).

Spices and Condiments in and Around Andhra Pradesh

R.Basavaraju

Spices and condiments are used as food adjuncts to add aroma, flavor and taste contain essential oils have nutritional and medicinal values, they are used whole, ground, paste or liquid form for flavoring and seasoning various types of food. Most spices increase the self life of the food, especially the dry varieties. Some are used to improve texture and some to introduce palatable colour or odour. An attempt has been made to give a picture of spices and condiments of Andhra Pradesh, classification, botany, production and uses of some important spices.

Introduction

Andhra Pradesh is the fifth largest state in India. It lies between 12 - 37 N Latitude and 76-46 E and 84-46 longitudes in southern part of India. The total area of the state is 2,75,068 sq. km. Topographically 35 % of the state area lies below 150m altitude forming coastal plains; about 15 % area lies between150-300m' 37 % area between 300-600m; 10 % area between 600-900m and the remaining area lies above 900m altitude. The state comprises of twenty three districts which are grouped into three distinct regions viz., Rayalaseema, Telangana and Coastal Andhra Pradesh. Geographically the state can be divided into coastal plains (Srikakulam to Nellore districts), Eastern Ghats running parallel to east coast and western pene-plains (covering Kurnool plains, most pats of Anatapur district and Telangana districts). About 64,000sq.Km of the total geographical area is under forests and 50 % of it covered in Eastern Ghats. The state has monsoon type of tropical climate. The mean annual temperature in summer varies between, 20 C to 41C and in winter ranging from 13 C to 32 C. The average annual rainfall is around 940 mm. The major type of soils in the state are red, black, deltaic alluvial and coastal alluvial. The important rivers in the state are Godavari, Krishna, Pennar and Tungabhadra.[1]

Plants are the source of organized systems of medicine. Out of 17,500 flowering plants reported from India, about 8000 plants are used in various systems of Indian medicine (Ayurveda 2351, Siddha 1785, Homoeo 506 and Unani 979). Murthy et al., have reported about 2531 flowering plants species from this state and they have listed about 365 medicinal plants.[2]

The Spices and condiments have played a vital role in all the civilizations of antiquity, in ancient India and China. The majority of spices originated in the Asiatic tropics and was among the first objects of commerce between East and West. The quest for spices was once a powerful force in world history. The spices cannot be grouped as foods, for they contain less nutritive value. However, they give good flavor and aroma to food and add greatly to the pleasure of eating. They stimulate the appetite and increase the secretion flow of gastric juices. For this reason they are commonly known as "food adjuncts". The aromatic value of the spices is due to the presence of the essential oils. In general, all aromatic vegetable products that are used for flavouring foods and drinks are known as spices. Condiments are spices or other flavouring substances which posses a sharp taste, and are commonly added to food after it has been cooked. According to the International Organization for standardization, there is no clear cut division between spices and condiments and so they are clubbed together. The term spices and condiments applies to such natural plant or vegetable products of mixtures thereof, in whole or ground form, as are used for imparting flavor, aroma and piquancy to and for seasoning food. Spices are mostly used as flavouring agents in a number of food products; such as curries, backery products, pickles, processed meats, beverages, liquors etc. They enhance or vary the flavor of foods, also flavor disguisers. Some spices possess antioxidant properties, while others are used as carminatives. Some spices are mainly used as preservatives in some foods like pickles and chutney. Others like clove and mustard possess strong anti-microbial properties and as such prevent food spoilage. Spices have been used since ages to preserve food specially meat and fish for long periods when there was no refrigeration. Many spices also possess important physiological and medicinal properties.[3,4]

Spices are obtained from a large number of different plants. They are parts of plant, such as roots, stems, leaves, buds, flowers, barks, fruits or seeds. Most of the spices owe their flavouring properties to volatile oils and in some cases to fixed oils and small amount of resins which are known as oleoresins. In many cases, no single compound is responsible for flavours, a blend of different compounds such as alcohols, esters, terpenes, organic acids, resins, alkaloids, and sulphur containing compounds contribute to the flavor. In addition all spices contain the usual components of plant products such as proteins, carbohydrates, fibre, minerals and tannins or polyphenols.[3]

There are about 70 species of spices grown in different parts of the world. Many of them are grown in our country India. Around 52 species have been identified by the Indian Spices Board till now. Classifying the spices and to propose strict demarcating lines among them is very difficult. All aromatic vegetables used for flavouring foods as per definition, can be classified under spices. Other people restrict the term spices to the hardened and preservable parts of the plant that are usually used in the powdered form.[4]

Classification of Spices:

Spices have been classified based on different parameters. However none of the classifications are mutually exclusive. Each of them either has some lacunae or overlapping. Some of the classifications are outlined below.

A. Based on plant part used as a spice

I. Roots:

II. Underground parts.

III. Bark

IV. Leaves

V. Inflorescence/flowers.

VI. Fruits

VII. Seeds

B. Based on botanical relationship

I. Apiaceae: Coriander, Cumin

II. Ceasalpinaceae: Tamarind

III. Fabaceae: Fenugrek

IV. Myrtaceae: Clove

V. Lauraceae: Tej pat

VI. Liliaceae: Garlic, Onion

VII. Piperaceae: Pepper

VIII. Rutaceae: Curry leaf

IX. Solanaceae: Chillies

X. Zingiberaceae: Ginger, Cordomom, Turmeric.

C. Based on longevity

I. Annual

II. Biennial

III. Perennial

D. Based on active component/characteristic features

I. Pungent spices: Pepper, Chilli, Ginger,Musterd etc

II. Aromatic fruits and seeds: Cardamom, Nutmeg etc.

III. Aromatic bark: Cinnamon, Cassia etc.

IV. Phenolic spices: Clove

V. Colouring spices: Saffron, Turmeric

VI. Umbelliferous fruits and seeds: Aniseed, Caraway, Celery, Coriander, Cumin etc.

E. Mixed classification

I. Major spices: Cardamom, Black pepper, Ginger, Turmeric

II. Seed spices: Corinader,Cumin,Fennel,Celery

III. Tree spices: Clove, Nutmeg, Cinnamom,Tamarind

IV. Herbal spices: Rosemary, Thyme,Parsley

V. Other spices: Vanilla, Saffron, Asafoetida, Garlic

Botany, Composition and uses of spices

Turmeric (*Curcuma longa* Linn. Zingiberaceae)

Turmeric is a tufty perennial herb about 1m.high. Rhizome thick much-branched, golden yellow. Leaves large, entire, long-sheathed, glabrous on both sides. Inflorescence cylindrical arising from the leaves, on a scape of yellow flowers and greenish or whitish bracts with pink tips. Extensively cultivated as a spice and medicinal plant.

Turmeric contains essential oil of around 5.8 % containing di-phellandrene, d-sabinene, cineol, borneol and zingiberene. It also contains compesterol, stigmasterol, cholesterol,monocyclic sesquilerpene, ketone,turmerone and p-totyl methyl carbinol and curcumin. Turmeric owes its colour primarily to curcuminoids ranging from 0.2 to 2 % depending on the species and on pre and post harvest factors. Turmeric is an important condiment used in cooking, specially in the form of curry powder. It also used in cosmetics and as natural dye for colouring wool, silk, cotton, confectionaries and in food industries. It is antiseptic and has antimicrobial properties. Curcumin is a antioxidant and can inhibit cancer. The pharmacological properties of curcumin includes anti-inflammatory, antioxidant, inhibition of platelet aggregation, local spasmolytic, hepatoprotective, and choleretic properties.[4,5]

Cardamom (*Elettaria cardamomum* Maton. Zingiberaceae)

A tall herbaceous perennial with subterranean branching root stock, 1.5 to 5 m in height; leaves subsessile, elliptic or lanceolate with sheathing base; flowers in panicle which are many for a plant arising from the base of the vegetative shoots, upright first and becoming prostrate, lip of the corolla white, streaked with violet, fruits trilocular, subglobose capsules, marked with many fine vertical ribs, seeds 15-20 per pod, brownish black covered by a thin mucilaginous membrane.

The principal constituents of volatile oil are cineol, myrcene, terinene, d-limonne, sabinene and terpineol acetate, sesquiterpenes, monoterpene hydrocarbons, 1,8-cineole, linaool acetate. The aqueous portion of the steam distillate contains 0.5 % essential oil and one of the chief constituents is borneol. The component fatty acids of the fixed oil is caprylic caproin, palmitic oleoic and linoleic acids.

Cardamon is mainly used as flavouring agent for sweets, beverages, sweetmeats, liquors and various bakery products. The oil from the seeds is used for treatment of inflammation of the eye lids. Cardamom is a carminative and is used together with betel leaves. The root and fruits of cardamom are used for its laxative and tonic properties. They are used as diuretic stimulant, stomachic and correcting menstrual disorders.[4,5]

Clove (*Syzygium aromaticum* (L.) Merrill & Perry Myrtaceae. Syn: *Eugenia aromaticum*)

A pyramidal or conical evergreen tree usually grows upto 12m in height with a single main stem bearing obliquely oriented branches, leaves simple, lanceolate, gland-dotted, fragrant; flower buds greenish to pink, clustered at the ends of the branches, highly aromatic; fruits fleshy, dark pink drupes, seeds oblong, grooved on one side.

Clove contains a heavy volatile oil of 16-20 %, a camphor resin 6 %, caryophylin and eugenin the alkaloids, woody fibre, gum etc. The main constituents of volatile oil are eugenol, eugenol acetate, caryophyliene, methyl n-amyl-carbinol, methyl furfural alcohol, dimethyl furfural, methyl-n-heptyl carbinol, naphthalene, and vanillin. Clove also contains calcium, phosphorus, iron, sodium, potassium, thamine, ribflovin, niacin and vitamin A & C. The clove buds, stem, and leaves on steam distillation yield substantial amounts of volatile oils. The bud contains free eugenol, eugenol acetate and caryopheline. The stem oil contains more free eugenol than bud oil, while the leaf oil contains least eugenol and eugenol acetate.

Clove is used either as whole or in powder form in preparing curry powder sauces, pickles, preservatives and ketch up. It is used for flavouring cakes, puddings, cookies, chocolate and candies. Clove oil is used in confectioneries. Besides being used in relieving toothache, headache and rheumatic pain. It has antiseptic, anti-inflammatory and analgesic properties. The oil used as carminative, spasmodic and aids digestion. It is now used in soaps, detergents and perfumery industries.[4,5]

Fennel (*Foenicum vulgare* Mill. Apiaceae)

An aromatic perennial herb 1-2 m high. Leaves alternate, 3 or 4 times pinnate, the ultimate leaflets very numerous, filiform, very elongated, the superior leaves with sheaths longer than the blade. Umbels compound, large, long-pedunculate, nearly regular. Flowers yellow, not invoucrate, calyx with 5 very slight teeth. Petals 5 entire,tips onvolute. Stamens 5, ovary 2- celled; stylopodium large, conical. Fruit avoid,6 mm long by 2 mm in diameter, greenish; glabrous mericarp compressed dorsally, semicylindrical, with 5 prominent, regular ribs. Seeds some what concave with longitudinal furrows. The fruit tastes sweet and pungent.

The mineral contents of fennel are calcium, phosphorous, iron, sodium, potassium and vitamin contents are thiamine, riboflavin, niacin, and vitamin-C. Its caloric value is 370.The composition of oil varies widely according to variety and origin. Indian fennel contains palmitic acid, petroselinic acid, d-pinene, camphene, d-phellendrene, limonene, anethole, anisaldehyde, p-ansic acid and dipentene d-fenchone. Methyl chavacol and foeniculin are also present as seed oils. The diuretic properties of fennel are attributed to the presence of glycolic acid.

Fennel is mostly used as flavouring agent in food. Young leaves of the tree are used raw or cooked with curry. The seeds are generally used for flavouring and fruit is commonly used as masticatory. The seed and oil has a variety of medicinal properties. The leaves of fennel are digestive, appetizing and stimulating. The seeds are sweet, laxative, aphrodiasic and arrest bleeding. The oil of fennel, distilled from the dry seeds is aromatic, carminative and antispasmodic. It is used in various carminative preparations.[4,5]

Ginger (*Zingiber officinale* Rosc. Zingiberaceae)

A slender, perennial rhizomatous herb; leaves linear, sessile glabrous; flowers yellowish green in oblong, cylindric spikes, ensheathed in a few scarious, glabrous bracts; fruits oblong capsules. The rhizomes are white to yellowish brown in colour, irregularly branched, somewhat annulated and laterally flattened. The growing tips are covered over by a few scales. The surface of the rhizome is smooth and if broken a few fibrous elements of the vascular bundles project out of the cut ends. Cultivated throughout India, run wild in some place in the Western ghats.

Ginger contains 1-3 % essential oil with a characteristic pleasant and aromatic odour. The major constituents are monoterpenes, sesquiterpenes, and oxygenated terpenes. The other constituents are chovicol, zingiberene, zingiberol, n-decylaldehyde, n-nonyaldehyde,d-camphene, methyl heptanone, cineole, d-borneol, geraneol, linaool, citral, nonanol, heptanes, octane gingediol, methylgediol and limonene. The non pungent principles are palmitic and other fatty acids while the pungent principles are oxymethyl phenols such as gingerol, shagoal, zingerone and related compounds.

Ginger is used in dried, preserved and green forms. Because of its pleasant aroma and pungency. It is widely used as flavouring agent in the preparation of various food products like ginger bread, confectioneries, curry powder, curried meats, pickles, and soft drinks like ginger cocktail, gingerella, and carbonated drinks like ginger beer. It is also used for preparation of oleoresins and essential oils. Ginger oil finds wide use in perfumery. It has a variety of medicinal properties and is used as antiinflamatory and digestive agents. It possesses anti-oxidant properties and may be added to edible oils and fats to protect them against rancidity. It is carminative, stimulant, and given for flatulence and colic. It has also hypoglycemic activity.[4,5]

Tejpat (*Cinnamomum tamala* Nees. Lauraceae)

A moderate sized evergreen tree 7.5 m in height with dark brown or blackish rough bark and pinkish or reddish brown blaze; leaves simple, opposite, sub-opposite or alternate, ovate-lanceolate or ovate–oblong, acuminate, coriaceous, glabrous, 3-nerved from base to apex; flowers pale yellowish in axillary and terminal, lax puberulous panicles; fruit ovoid, fleshy, black drupe, supported by enlarged perianth tube.

It is a flavouring agent. The flavor is because of an alcohol soluble essential oil containing 70-80 % cinnamic aldehyde. Moreover, high amounts of d-phellandrene and eugenol are found among other constituents. Besides flavouring agent, tejpat oil is used for perfuming soap and in medicines. It is used for treatment of boils, conjunctivitis, itching, diarrhea, fatigue, tiredness and urinary problems.[4,5]

Corinader (*Coriandrum sativum* Linn. Apiaceae)

A glabrous, aromatic, herbaceous annual 30-90 cm in height, leaves decompound, lower ones long-petioled and upper ones short-petioled or subsessile, imparipinnatisect into linear-setaceous lobes. Flowers small, white or pinkish purple in compound terminal umbels; fruits yellowish brown, globular and ribbed, separating into two halves (mericarps) each containing a seed.

It yields a colour less pale yellow oil, chief constituent of which is cinnamaldehyde, eugenol, benzaldehyde, methyl-amyl n-amyl ketone, rutin, linaqalool, d-z-pinene, dl-z pinene, p-cymene, dipentene, y-terpinene, phellandrene, terpinolene, and traces of coriandrinol, angelicin, l-borneol,n-decyoladehyde thymol, elemol, geraniol caryophyllene, safrole, cinamyl alcohol, methyleugenol.

The constituent fatty acids of the oil are palmitic, petrosebinic linolic acids. Besides variety of minerals and vitamins, coriander contains high amount of vitamin A.

Coriander fruits are used as culinary preparations, flavouring liquors, cocoa preparations and in confectionery. It has medicinal properties and used for the treatment of bronchial asthma, bronchitis, small pox, and conjunctivitis. Coriander leaves are stimulant, and tonic. Coriander bark oil has high germicidal activity and is used as fungicide.[4,5]

Asafoetida (*Ferula asafoetida* Linn. Apiaceae)

A herbaceous perenninal with fleshy, massive carrot-shaped root with one or more forks, stem1.8 to 3 m high, solid, clothed with membranous leaf sheaths; leaves radical, 45 cm long, shiny coriaceous with pinnatifid segments and channeled petiode; flowers 10-20 in the main and 5-6 in the partial umbels; fruits flat, thin reddish brown.

The major constituents of asafoetida are moisture, ash, resin, gum glucuronic acid, galactose, arabinose, rhamnose. Volatile oil is 10-17 %, essential oil 6-10 % containing sulfur compounds, umbelliferone, ferulic acid and pinene. Recently, phellopterin, isopimpinellin and byakagelicin have been isolated.

It is used as a medicine and as a condiment. The gum resin possesses antispasmodic, carminative, expectorant and stimulant properties. It is effective in curing respiratory problems, and cold attacks. It is used for treating hysteria, syphilis, excessive flatulence and bronchitis. It has antimicrobial properties. Essential oil shows protective action against fat induced increase in plasma fibrinogen and decease in coagulation time and fibrinolytic activity an alimentary hyperlipaemia.[4,5]

Fenugreek (*Trigonella foenum-graecum* Linn. Fabaceae)

An aromatic, erect annual, 30-60 cm in height; leaves pinnate,3-foliate,leaflets toothed; flowers white or yellowish white, axillary; fruits pods , 5-7.5 cm long with long persistent beak; seeds 10-20 per pod, greenish brown along with a deep groove across one cornered.

It contains fatty acids, an alkaloid trignelline and a liquid base choline. The saponins of trigonella contain sapogenin, diosgenin, gitogenin, tigogenin, reotigogenin, yanogenin. The non saponificable fraction contains carotene, ergosterol and phospholipids, while saponifiable fraction contains a nonphenolic lactating factor. The alcoholic extracts of the plant also contains a high amount of an amino acid cystein. Glycosides, graecunines, fenugrin B, etc are also present in the seeds.

Fenugreek is used to increase the flow of milk of cattles as it contains a lactation promoting factor. Used to cure fatigue, small pox, gastric troubles, gout, flatulence, loss of appetite, irregular period in women and sexual weakness. It is also used in colic flatulence, dysentery, diarrhea, chronic cough, enlargement of spleen and liver, rickets and diabetes. Fenugreek reduces blood sugar levels in diabetic patients. It contains diogenin which is used as starting material in synthesis of sex hormones and oral contraceptives. It is often grounded and mixed with cotton seeds and fed to the cattles for increase in milk production.[4,5]

Garlic (*Allium sativum* Linn. Liliaceae)

An annual glabrous, bulbous herb, with pungent odour. Bulb short, consists of several smaller bulbs (called cloves) and is surrounded by a thin, white or pinkish sheath. Leaves flat and narrow, attenuated at the apex, nerves parallel. Flowers white or pink with bulbils in globose head covered with a large bract. Cultivated all over the country.

Allylprophudisulphide, responsible for the smell, is the main constituent of essential oil of garlic. Other constituents of the oil are diallysulphide and two more sulphur containing compounds. Allicin, allisatin -I, allisatin-II, are the chief plant antibiotics obtained from it. Allicin is obtained from alline by the action of the enzyme allianase. Allythiamin has been isolated from the bulbs of garlic. The carbohydrates in garlic bulb consist mainly of invertase and polyfructodase.

Garlic is used for flavouring curries, chutnies, soaps and stews. It also contains a variety of medicinal properties. It acts as stimulant, carminative, emmenagogue, antirheumatic, antihelinthic. It is also used as a vermifuge i.e. to expel worms, specially round worms. Garlic is known to lower cholesterol in the blood and is recommended for heart diseases and arteriosclerosis. Garlic also shows antibacterial and anti-fungal effects against a variety of strains. It has anti-inflammatory activity and is effective in the treatment of rheumatoid arthritis. It is also hepato-protective.

Pepper (*Piper longum* Linn. Piperaceae)

A slender sub-scandent herb, branches erect, straggling or sometimes climbing, hairless, with swollen nodes and those of creeping branches with roots at lower nodes. Leaves alternate, variable in shape usually egg-shaped-heart –shaped, 7-15x 4-6 cm, base heart-shaped and unequal, apex acute to acụminate, margin entire, hairless. Male spikes erect, 2-7 cm long, greenish yellow, fleshy, cylindrical, with minute male flowers. Female spikes erect, 1-3 cm long, yellow. Fruiting spikes cylindrically oblong. Berries globose, about 2mm across, partly sunken in the rachis, compactly arranged red turning black when ripe.

It contains a volatile oil, resin and an alkaloid piperine. The essential oil consists of alpha-pinene, beta-pinene, 1-alpha-phellandrene, di-limonene, piperonal, dihydrocarveol, alpa - caryophllene and piperidine complex. The oleoresin contains piperine,chavacine, other piperidides pipercides and piperidine. The volatile alkaloid alpha-methyl pyrroline is also present.

Pepper is indispensible in sauces, soups, condiments, pickles and for seasoning various types of dishes. It is stimulant, pungent, aromatic, digestive, and appetizer. It increases flow of saliva and gastric juices and used for digestive disorders. Piperidine, piperine is a potent anti-inflammatory agent and pepper is used for gum inflammation, toothache, muscular pain. It is also potent analgesic.[4,5]

Chilli (*Capsicum annuum* Linn. Solanaceae)

A herbaceous, short- lived perennial, upto 1 m in height; leaves oblong, glabrous; flowers solitary, rarely in pairs white to bluish white, berries green, maturing into yellow then to red, seeds white or cream to yellow , thin, almost circular, having long placental connections.

Chilli gives a fatty oil (9-13 %) and on steam distillation gives volatile oil (0.16 – 39 %). Chilli contains pungent principle capsaicinoids that is a mixture of capsaicin, dihydro capsaicin, homo-capsaicin, non-hydrocapsaicin, and homo-dihydrocapsaicin. Some pigments like capsanthin, capsorubin, zeaxanhin, lutein, cryptoxanthin, and xanthophylls are also present. Chilli is rich in vitamin C. Seed oil contains citro-stadienol, gramisterol, methyllophenol, ethylphenol, lophenol, cycloeucalenol, obtusterol etc.

The green chillies are used fresh for garnishing or flavouring savory dishes. Bell pepper or capsicum is extensively used as food flavouring in processed foods, meat and vegetable soups. Dry chilli is extensively used in curry powder and curried dishes. Capsaicin is a potent anti-inflammatory and analgesic agent. Chilli is used for treatment of headaches, toothaches, muscular sprains, low backache and sciatic pain. It has cholesterol lowering effects and is used as anti-obesity agent. It is also digestive and increases saliva flow. Chilli also has potent anti-microbial properties.[4,5]

Tamarind (*Tamarindus indica* Linn. Caesalpiniaceae)

A large to very large evergreen tree upto 30 m in height with dark grey bark having longitudinal fissures and deep cracks; leaves paripinnate upto 15 cm long, rachis slender, channeled, leaflets 10-20 pairs, subsessile, oblong; flowers yellow, striped with red in laxz, few flowered racemes at the ends of the branchlets; fruits pods, brownish ash coloured, slightly curved, subcompressed, with a shallow oblong pit on each side of the flat faces; seeds enveloped by a toughy leathery membrane(the endocarp) and pulpy mesocarp, tests shining, hard. Tamarind trees are present throughout India, particularly in the South India, often cultivated.

Fruits contain traces of oxalic acid while seeds contain a fatty oil. The pectin contains polysaccharides and xylon. The pulp contains tartaric acid and other acids. Leaves contain flavonoid glycosides saponaretin, vitexin, orientin and homoorientin. Hordenine isolated from leaves, bark and flowers.

The root bark is astringent constipating, emmenagogue and tonic and is useful in diarrhea, asthma, amenorrhoea, singivitis and ulcers. The leaves are sour, astringent, thermogenic, anthelmintic, anodyne, anti-inflammatory, antifungal, diuretic, febrifuge, aperients and ophthalmic. The fruits are sour, sweet, refrigerant, digestive, carminative, laxative, antiseptic and febrifuge. The seeds astringent, cooling, stomachic. Tamarind is used as an acidulant in some food preparations. It is digestive, antiflatulent, cooling laxative, and antiseptic. Tamarind pulp being rich in vitamin C is prescribed in scurvy, common cold and fevers. It is used in dyeing, tanning, and polishing and cleaning metalware. Tamarind powder finds extensive use as a sizing material in textile industry.[4,5]

Onion (*Allium cepa* Linn. Liliaceae)

A biennial or perennial herb with aromatic fleshy underground bulb; leaves linear, hollow, cylindric and fleshy; flowers many white in globular umbels, spathe composed of 2-3 reflexed walls. The underground bulbs which are medicinally used vary in size, colour, shape, firmness, strength of flavor and keeping quality. Onions are cultivated throughout India.

The chief constituent of the essential oil is allyl propyl disulphide. The volatile oil contains methanol, propionaldehyde, n-propyl-thiol hydrogen sulphide, acetaldehyde an-hydroxy propanthiol, 4-hexenyl aldehyde, cyclo-allin and alpha-glutamyl peptides-(1-proponyl)-cysteine sulphoxide is considered very important.

Fresh onions have a strong anti-microbial effect. Onions offer a considerable relief in neuralgia, headaches and migrane. It is also useful in dyspepsia or mild indigestion and induces appetite in food, removes common cold, overcome flatulence and improves digestion. Onions are found beneficial in inflammation, ulceration of mouth and gums and toothache. It is used in gout, constipation and urinary disorders.[4,5]

Cumin (*Cuminum cyminum* Linn. Apiaceae)

A slender annual herb, leaves twice or thrice 3-partite segments filiform. Inflorescence umbels compound, bacts and bracteoles present, fruit cylindric, tip narrowed primary ridges filiform, distinct, secondary usually hispidulous. Cumin is cultivated all over India.

Seeds yield a volatile oil with an unpleasant bitter taste containing cuminaldeyde, p-cymene, pines, cuminyl alcohol, phellandrene and l-terpineol. Moreover, glucosides of luteolin, apigenin and d-manitol are present in the seeds.

It is generally used as an additive in increasing flavor of different food preparations. It also has a variety of medicinal properties and used as carminative, astringent, stomachic and useful in dyspepsia and diarrhea. The oil of cumin is used to flavor curries and other culinary preparations, confectionery, beverages, liqueurs and caridals.[4,5]

Curry Leaf (*Murraya koenigii* Linn.Spren.gel. Rutaceae)

An aromatic shrub or small tree; leaves pinnate, leaflets mostly ovate, crenate-dentate; flowers white in corymbose cymes; berries purplish black. Present throughout India, often cultivated.

Leaves and fruits contain alkaloids koenimbine, mahanimbine and koenigicine. Moreover, leaves contain mahanibidine, cyclomahanimbin curryangine andcurryanine. Marrayanine, mukoeic acid and girinimbine were also obtained from the bark. Curry leaves contain moisture 66.3 %, protein 6.1 %, fat 1.0 %, carbohydrates 16.0 %, fibre 6.4 % and mineral matter 4.2 % per 100 grams. The leaves are rich in calcium, phosphorous, iron, nicotinic acid and vitamin C. The leaves also contain a residual glucoside named koenigin.

The leaves are extensively used for flavouring curries, chutneys, soups, pickles etc. Curry leaves possess the function of stomachic and is also mild laxative. It is used in the treatment of morning sickness, nausea, flatulence and vomiting. It is a hair tonic and is considered beneficial in preventing premature graying of hair. The aqueous extract of leaves on oral administration has been shown to give hypoglycemic activity in normal and alloxan diabetic dogs.

Wild relatives are an important genetic resource on which the sovereign rights exist for a country in the post CBD (Convention on Biological Diversity) regime. There exists a tremendous potential for utilization of the wild gene pool by incorporation of genes against biotic /abiotic stresses and for enhancing yield and productivity in crop species. A total of 22 related species belonging to genera Capsicum, Piper, Cinnamomum, Curcuma, Eugenia, Murraya, Vanilla, Zingiber, and Pimpinella represent the wild relatives of chillies, pepper, cinnamon, turmeric, clove, curry leaf, vanilla, ginger, aniseed are represented in Andhra Pradesh (Pandravada, Sivaraj, Kamala, Suniland Varaprasad,2008). One species of Capsicum frutecens is reported from the tribal pockets of north coastal region and Kurnool districts. Under pepper, four species of *Piper attenuatum, P. hymenophyllum, P. longum, and P. nigrum* are reported from Eat Godavari, Visakhapatnam, Vizianagaram, Kurnool, Chittoor and Khammam districts. Under turmeric, four species *Curcuma aromatica, C. decipiens, C. neilgherrensis, and C. psedomontana* are reported from north coastal and north Telangana regions, Chittoor and Mahaboobnagar districts. Under ginger, four species *Zingiber capitatum, Z. purpureum, Z. roseum and Z. wifhtianum* are reported from East Godavari, Visakhapatnam, Warangal and Mahaboobnagar districts.[6]

Production of Spices

India is the foremost country in production, consumption and export of spices. Blessed with tropical, sub-tropical and temperate climates and varied soil types make India possible to grow almost all spices. Every state and Union territory grows at least a few spices. Andhra Pradesh, Karnataka, Kerala, Gujarat, Madhya Pradesh, Maharashtra, Orissa, Rajasthan, Tamil Nadu, and West-Bengal are the leading spice producing states. Total production of spices in India during 2002-2003 was 30.31 lakh tones from an area of 25.36 lakh hectares. Production has increased to 46.64 lakh tones from an area of 26.49 lakh hectares during 2006-2007.

India is the largest producer and supplier of Turmeric in the world, where it was grown in an area of 183917 hectares, producing annually 856464 tones during 2006-2007. In India, Andhra Pradesh is the leading state, where it was grown in an area of 64500 hactares producing 400920 tones during 2006-2007.

India has become the world's largest producer of Chilli since last many years. Chilli was cultivated in 827950 hectares, producing 906994 tones in 2002-2003, there was increase in the production upto 1325273 tones in 2006-2007, covering an area of 809437 hectares in our country. Andhra Pradesh stands first in the production of chilli, where the production was 766000 tones in 2006-2007, covering an area of 214000 hectares. In 2007-08 exports of chillies reached a record level of 2.09 lakh tones valued at Rs 1097.50 crores, accounting for a share of 47 percent in volume and 25 percent in value of the total export of spices and spices products from India.

India is the largest producer of ginger contributing over 30% of the world production. All India report of ginger production show's Ginger production was 422820 tones, in the area of 103220 hectares during 2002-2003. The yield has shown increase in the production to 721530 tones, covering an area of 129014 hectares. The contribution of Andhra Pradesh was 3310 tones, in the area of 2030 hectares during 2002-2003, which has increased to 10300 tones during 2006-2007, in the area of 2430 hectares.

India has premier position for the supply of Coriander to the world market. In India coriander was cultivated in the area of 302450 hectares, with production of 188950 tones in 2002-2003. The cultivation spread to 361767 hectares to increase the yield to 287647 tones during 2006-2007. The contribution of A.P. was 10060 tones from the area of 25380 hectares, in 2006-2007.

In India Tamarind was cultivated in the area of 61958 hectares, producing 178994 tones during 2002-2003. The production increased to 190073 tones covering an area of 58042 hectares in the year 2006-2007. The contribution of A.P. was 13405 tones in

2002-2003, which increased to 19483 tones during the year 2006-2007.

Andhra Pradesh is one of the major spices producing States in India with its major share in the production of chillies, turmeric, and tamarind. The State contributes to nearly 30 percent of the total spice production in the country. Considering the Importance of the Andhra Pradesh in spices trade, the Spices Board has initiated many programmes. They are:Quality improvement programmes, Supply of polythene sheets to farmers for drying of chillies and turmeric under hygienic conditions, Training programmes for farmers, Training progammes for officials of the State Agric/ Horticulture departments, Setting up of Spices Park in Guntur, Setting up of Quality Evaluation Lab for spices in Guntur, Campaign in major chilli growing districts-Guntur, Prakasam, Warangal, and Khammom-to educate growers on the need to improve post harvest practices. [7]

References

1. Ravi Prasad Rao, B, M.Sridhar Reddy and T. Pullaiah. Flora and vegetation of Andhra Pradesh, Proceedings of Andhra Pradesh Akademi of Sciences (Special Issue), 12:1-13. (2008).
2. G.V.S Murthy,. J.H.F Benjamin and Bir Bahadur.. Medicinal plants of Andhra Pradesh, Proceedings of Andhra Pradesh Akademi of Sciences (Special Issue), 12: 122-137. (2008).
3. B.P. Pandey, Economic Botany, Spices and Condiments, S.Chand & Company Ltd. New Delhi, 283-344. (2007).
4. Amit Krishna De. Recent Trends in Spices and Medicinal Plants Research, Associated Publishing Company, New Delhi.1-18, (2000).
5. N.P Prajapathi,., S.S Purohit,., A.K Sharma,. and T Kumar., A Hand Book Of Medicinal Plants. A Complete Source Book, Agrobios (India), 183-202. (2004).
6. S.R Pandravada,., N.Sivaraj, , V.Kamala, N.Sunil, and K.S. Varaprasad, Genetic resources of wild relatives of crop plants in Andhra Pradesh-Diversity, Distribution and Conservation, Proceedings of Andhra Pradesh Akademi of Sciences (Special Issue), 101-119. (2008).
7. SPICE BOARD of India web site: www.indianspices.com